D0097057

Everything Changes

The Insider's Guide to
Cancer in Your 20s and 30s

Kairol Rosenthal

WILEY

John Wiley & Sons, Inc.

Published by John Wiley & Sons, Inc., Hoboken, New Jersey
Published simultaneously in Canada

For general information about our other products and services, please contact our Customer Care Department within the United States at (800) 762-2974, outside the United States at (317) 572-3993 or fax (317) 572-4002.

Wiley also publishes its books in a variety of electronic formats. Some content that appears in print may not be available in electronic books. For more information about Wiley products, visit our web site at www.wiley.com.

Library of Congress Cataloging-in-Publication Data:
Rosenthal, Kairol, date.
    Everything changes : the insider's guide to cancer in your 20s and 30s / Kairol Rosenthal.
        p.   cm.
    Includes bibliographical references and index.
    ISBN 978-0-470-29402-4 (pbk.)
        1. Cancer—Popular works.   2. Young adults—Diseases.   I. Title.
    RC263.R645   2009
    616.99'4—dc22
                                                                    2008049900

Printed in the United States of America

10   9   8   7   6   5   4   3   2   1

Contents

Acknowledgments

From activism to learning how to build support, to enacting healthcare policy, the cancer community owes a hefty thanks to the AIDS community for paving the way. I owe special thanks to editor Michael Denneny, whose trailblazing work in publishing the first books on HIV and AIDS cleared a path for a book such as this. I am grateful for his personal support of my project; his editorial eyes on my early manuscript were instrumental in bringing this book to fruition. Thank you to my tenacious agent, Regina Ryan, who is a champion of books that make a difference, and to my editor, Christel Winkler, who had her antennae up and knew that a book on young adult cancer needed to be written even before we met. I'm most appreciative to production editor Rachel Meyers at Wiley and freelance copy editor Patricia Waldygo for their eagle-eyed editing skills. I also want to thank my other "in-house" editor, Shannon Fisk, who gave endless close readings of this work.

I am especially grateful to the twenty-five men and women in this book who gave me carte blanche to reveal bits and pieces of their lives as I saw fit. I would not have found these cancer patients without the help of the following individuals and institutions: the Charlotte Maxwell Complementary Clinic, Beverly Lowe, Women's Cancer Resource Center, Margo Rivera-Weiss, Celeste Whitewolf, the Ida and Joseph Friend Cancer Resource Center, Mimi Roth, the University of Alabama Kirkland Clinic, Erin Street, and Lydia Cheyne. I wish to thank Craig Newmark for creating Craigslist .org, which connected me to many of the patients in this book and to volunteer transcriptionists. I extend a gracious thank you to these volunteers: Maya Nikin, Ellen Seremet, Laura Sciortino, Karleen Chong, Lindsay Baker, Sheri Martin, Claire Rasmussen, Elizabeth Kowlaski, Amy Schoenhals, Lori Ann Spencer, Rachel Lukasavige, Jennifer Buzick, and Janelle Sosh. Thanks also to photographers Andrew Young and Michelle Kondracki, whose photos appear on the cover.

The following individuals have dedicated their careers to furthering the young adult cancer cause, and I thank them for sharing their expertise with me: Heidi Adams, Dr. Archie Bleyer, Dr. Leonard Sender, Page Tolbert, and Brad Zebreck, as well as the many experts who contributed information to the resource sections of this book. Librarians Mary Pranica and Scott Thomson from the Lurie Cancer Center, Campaign for Better Health Care, and the reference staff of the Evanston Public Library have lent hours of research assistance, for which I thank them.

I am especially thankful to Jana Vitols, Lisa Friedman, Emily Fox, Heather Phillips, Sara Braun, Lowell Brown, Chris Howland, Barbara Flood, Max Raimi, Karin Steinbrueck, Daniel Biss, Nate Burbank, and Asimina Chremos for their brainstorming, inquiry, and interest in this book. And to my extended Rosenthal, Arnheim, and Cohen family, for their continual enthusiasm about this project.

I thank the City of Chicago Department of Cultural Affairs and the Illinois Arts Council for their partial support of this project through a Community Arts Assistance Program grant.

Introduction

It is not the nitty-gritty details of how we were diagnosed or what treatments we are taking that interest me as much as what we do with our lives after the big cancer bomb is dropped in our laps. How do we think about life when we are facing death? Nonetheless, I will give you the pithy lowdown on what was happening in my life when I was twenty-seven years old, so that you can better understand who I am and why I bothered to write this book.

At twenty-seven years old, I was brimming with the muse and confusion. I lived alone in a dilapidated three-story walk-up near the foot of the Bay Bridge in San Francisco. Working at under-the-table and menial nonprofit jobs, I had a minuscule income and shoddy health insurance. I wrote stories on my fire escape until three in the morning and was sending off manuscripts, applying to graduate school, choreographing performances, and penny pinching. I was single, dating, and sleeping around. My friends were trust-fund kids, dot-com geniuses, and receptionists, and one even traded blowjobs for rent. As I was determined to find a respectable and engaging day job, my schemes for how to support myself changed weekly.

I had long thought that chiropractors were quacks; if they gave you one wrong crack, you ended up a spoon-fed paraplegic for life. But after wrenching my neck in dance rehearsal, I was in pain, and a friend who was a receptionist at a chiropractor's office slipped me into the doctor's schedule. After five seconds on the table, the chiropractor pulled me to my feet and hauled me in front of her mirror. She pointed to a lump on my neck, demanding, "How long has this been here?" The lump was huge, and I was stunned that I had never noticed it. She ousted my friend from the front desk and sat me down in her swivel chair. We fished through the deck of ragged business cards in my wallet, searching for the I.D. card from my bottom-of-the-barrel health insurance company. She made me call the insurance company to demand an appointment that afternoon for blood work and chest X-rays. She then packed up my belongings and ushered me out the door.

As I quickly trekked up steep San Francisco hills on my way to the BART station, everything around me melted into vivid slow motion and I felt an immaculate weightlessness I had never experienced before. It was the absence of longing and wishing. The absence of regret and fear. I realized that I could evaporate right there on the sidewalk and leave the world knowing that my life had been complete. Perhaps I'm not twenty-seven, I thought. Perhaps I'm seventy-two in disguise. I scrambled down the escalator to the train. Okay, one regret: if this is cancer, I want to stay alive long enough to get a dog.

My insurance granted me a series of ten-minute urgent-care appointments with four different doctors who declared that I had a cold, allergies, or swollen glands. Despite my extreme fear of doctors and my instantaneous loathing of the medical system, I hacked through the red tape of my big-box, managed-care facility and obtained a botched biopsy, which came back negative. Six months later, my employer, who had been unable to recruit high-level staff due to the company's abysmal insurance coverage, switched to an HMO that allowed me to choose from a pool of doctors. I received an accurate diagnosis of stage II thyroid cancer that had metastasized to nineteen lymph nodes. I have since learned that many cancer patients in their twenties and thirties are diagnosed at more progressed stages of cancer, both because our symptoms are frequently dismissed by doctors and because we often do not have access to health insurance.

When I woke up the morning after my diagnosis, my first thought was the opposite of "Why me?" Why not me? Why a fifty-five-year-old truck driver, a nine-year-old in a pediatric unit, or my seventy-seven-year-old grandmother? Of course, me. Why the hell *not* me? This life is breakable, and I'm no more immune to pain and suffering than the next person. As I lay with my feet tangled in the covers, eighteen hours after receiving my diagnosis, cancer was not a shock. It was simply a continuum in learning that alongside pleasure and joy, life sometimes sucks. My summation was that anyone who dares to construe pain and injury as a personal affliction, rather than a human condition, hasn't been living with his or her eyes open. With that, I climbed out of bed and put one foot in front of the other.

When I divulged my diagnosis to other people, their eyes bugged out and their voices filled with disbelief. "You're too young," they replied. I agreed with a simple nod but wanted to blurt out, "No one is too young for cancer. I'm not an anomaly. Get over it. It could happen to you, too." In my mind, I silently defended the brutal reality that the person to whom I was speaking was no more impervious to death than I was; he or she just had the luxury of not having to think about it.

During my first months of cancer, my mail carrier got clever, finding new ways to lodge stacks of get-well cards and books into my slender mailbox. I thumbed through the cancer memoirs sent by my East Coast friends and family. Their pink covers were a mocking reminder that I should feel part of a community of survivors who describe their experiences as a fight and speak in optimistic and hopeful catchphrases that are ripe for talk shows and T-shirts. I felt like a freak compared to the patients in these books, not because they were often decades older than me, but because they made cancer sound like a ladies-who-lunch club. According to them, I was supposed to feel hopeful instead of desperate, quietly contemplative instead of loudly interrogative, and grateful to the cancer community instead of outraged at the healthcare system. On the inside jacket, their short bios read, "Such and such lives in Manhattan with her loving husband and their dogs." I was juggling multiple casual relationships, hoping to find someone who would hold me in his arms at night and dissolve my cancer fear. I was shamefully jealous of these women, their husbands, and their dogs.

In my first six months of living with cancer, I received enough phone numbers of friends of friends with cancer to fill a small Rolodex. Picking up the phone and calling a complete stranger, twice my age, with cancer was just as appealing to me as calling the nice, single Jewish boy whose mother had met my mother at synagogue. It wasn't going to happen. Between my rounds of treatment, I intermittently attended a monthly young adult cancer support group, where the atmosphere vacillated between relaxed and rigid. At times, I spoke freely, but most often I felt inhibited complaining about my stage II cancer while sitting next to a woman on the verge of hospice and across from a guy who had just lost a lung. I found I could unleash my feelings more easily by talking to my close friends who did not have cancer than to a room full of eight strangers who did.

A year and a half after my diagnosis, my friend Jenny introduced me to the first committed boyfriend I had during cancer. He was a painter who was simultaneously supportive of me and resentful and whiny when my treatment schedule and side effects pulled him away from his easel. He grew up in the Midwest and was eager to return there.

State disability, savings, and frugality had sustained me for almost two years, but I could no longer afford cancer in the rapidly gentrifying Bay Area. I was enticed by low rent and the idea of living closer to my family in Pittsburgh, so I moved with him to Chicago. Not surprisingly, we broke up one month after our arrival. Being unable to hack the smoke-saturated bars that were a cornerstone of Midwestern social life, I met few people, and my bed had an empty space for the first time in my cancer career.

My case had originally been billed as very treatable but was becoming much more complicated; suspicious new nodes appeared with every scan of my neck. A social butterfly from birth, I ached for the comfort of my San Francisco friends, yet I began to notice that two years of cancer had made an indelible mark on my capacity to endure solitude. During a long, freezing first winter in Chicago, I began to enjoy the anonymity of life in my basement apartment, in a city of three million people where no one knew me as "the dancer with cancer."

At a young adult cancer support group in Chicago, I sat every Tuesday night with eight women who chatted for an hour and a half about shopping and swimwear. It was the closest I'd ever come to attending a sorority party. I felt profoundly alone when interacting with these women and experienced more candor, understanding, and fun with the ex-offenders who were clients at my day job. I sat in church basements with rapists and murderers (a remarkably respectful and nice bunch of guys) teaching résumé writing and feeding them the organization's line that if you work hard enough, you can achieve anything. These men and I knew this was bullshit, that life's circumstances don't necessarily comply with will or effort.

My cancer was often pronounced by others as a creative blessing in disguise. "This is the content for your next performance. How healing and cathartic," they would exclaim. For me, choreography was art, not therapy. With a long list of subject matter that fascinated me, the last thing I wanted was cancer following me into the studio.

I worked alone in the studio for six months, and as fiercely as I resisted, I could not shake from my mind sets constructed of wheeled carts, costumes of sterile blue fabric, movements executed from lying down as if in bed, and phrases that emerged from relentless pacing and waiting. I planned to interview other young adults living with cancer and translate their words into movement images and sound scores. An extensive printed program would be for sale in the lobby, detailing their lives.

I became obsessed with the idea of interviewing twenty- and thirtysomething cancer patients for my performance and I began to reflect on my conversations with Seth, a thirty-three-year-old performance artist with lymphoma whom I met backstage after a show when I lived in San Francisco. We recognized each other's names through mutual friends and began to talk about our experiences living with cancer. The night we met, he and I spent five hours immersed in conversation. We were free from the constraints of a support group and had no need to speak politely. We weren't concerned with giving equal airtime to anyone besides the two of us. With no therapist or organizer present, I asked him blunt and personal questions that I wouldn't dare ask in a group. We continued to meet for dinners and talked on the phone. No cancer subject was off limits; we talked about our sex drives, partners, parents, loneliness, frustration, and our overly hormonal, racing minds that made us feel as if we were wired on speed.

Sets, costumes, and choreography receded into the background of my project, and simple, one-on-one conversations with young cancer patients became my focus; I was no longer crafting a performance but instead writing this book. Friends and family donated money for audio-recording equipment, and I received a travel grant from the City of Chicago Department of Cultural Affairs. I networked with social workers, posted on Craigslist, and sent out flyers that hung on church and Laundromat bulletin boards across the country. E-mails and calls from young adult cancer patients began flowing in.

I had lived with cancer for three years before learning that 70,000 young adults in their twenties and thirties are diagnosed with cancer in the United States every year. With this many young cancer patients sniffing anesthesia in operating rooms, absorbing beams of radiation, and sitting in chemo chairs across the country, I was astounded that I and so many others felt so alone. I discovered that other young adult cancer patients wanted to share with me in intimate conversation what they were not willing to reveal in support groups, what they would not tell their doctors or therapists, and what they had a difficult time saying to their friends and family.

While writing this book, I hung above my desk a quote from the closing scene in *The Breakfast Club*, where the geek played by Anthony Michael Hall writes in a letter to the principal, Mr. Vernon, "You see us as you want to see us, in the simplest terms, in the most convenient definitions." The "survivorship experience" has become a cultural phenomenon that is used to advance our disease on a national political level, to increase awareness, and to rally for needed psychosocial support services. Survivorship stories have also created a stereotype of cancer patients—even young adult cancer patients. We are seen as vocal, outspoken, sassy, sexy, insightful, spiritual, grateful, and empowered. By writing this book, I aspired to rip young adult cancer patients from the confines of these limited descriptors and perceptions. I wanted to reveal who we are, not in simple definitions but in the complexities of our real daily lives: what we think about while lying in bed at night; what we wish we could tell our lovers but are too afraid to; the ways in which we feel vulnerable, tender, and utterly uncertain what to do with ourselves; the times when cancer is not a fight but just a hard circumstance with which to live. I wanted to do this for the reader but also for myself. My friends and family were incredible, but I yearned for a level of understanding I had not found elsewhere.

Through these intimate conversations, young adult cancer patients revealed who they are as people, not only as survivors. For this reason,

I have chosen not to use the word *survivor* to describe them in the book. The word *patient* is an imperfect substitute, with its cold and clinical feel, but is more accurate than *survivor*, which many of the cancer patients I interviewed, myself included, did not accept as a label.

Over the course of three years, I have had twenty-five conversations with young adult cancer patients ages twenty to thirty-nine. Traveling throughout the United States to meet these strangers in person allowed for eye contact; extended silences; introductions to friends, roommates, and family; and sometimes the peeling away of clothing to reveal abdominal, chest, and neck scars. Face-to-face conversation was paramount in creating intimacy, which we often achieved within as little as half an hour after meeting.

I allowed conversations to simply unfold, rather than leading them with a prescribed list of questions. Since I'd undergone treatment, my mind had become a sieve. It was frustrating when questions slipped from my brain before I could ask them, but losing ourselves in the tangled mess of our minds led us to subjects and memories that would have been overlooked in a narrow question-and-answer format.

In these recorded conversations, I was seeking material that I could use to compile the antithesis of a patient memoir. I wanted the raw, confessional talk that spills out when one is not conscious of portraying an image on the page, is unconcerned with chronology and medical details, and is not trying to educate, prove a point, or sway the reader's mind. Orchestrating these more intentional aspects of the book was my job, which occurred when I sat down with the transcripts late at night and often months after the actual meetings took place.

I had recordings of twenty-five conversations lasting from three to ten hours each, so paying for professional transcription was unaffordable. I posted on Craigslist for volunteer transcriptionists and received so many responses I had to turn people away. Many of the volunteers who worked on these tediously long transcriptions had lost someone important to cancer, knew a young adult living with cancer, or were taking premed classes and wanted to immerse themselves in the world of cancer care. Without their help, this book would not exist.

Transcripts ranged from 40 to 120 pages apiece. In cutting away reams of text, I made sure that my allegiance remained with the reader; I have omitted details of stories that these patients would have chosen to include were they writing their own memoirs. A few patients used pseudonyms, and nearly all had told me details about ex-boyfriends or ex-girlfriends, family members, coworkers, or their doctors that they were eager to unload in conversation but asked that I not allow to be published. I have, of course, met their wishes, no matter how juicy or fantastic the story. I have reordered their words and sentences to make the conversations flow more smoothly on the page and added words where clarification was needed. Throughout this editing process I have worked painstakingly to maintain the patients' intentions and meaning.

I created sections for resources to save patients the chore of reinventing the research wheel. Focusing on issues that are most relevant to young adults, I have included only resources that I found most useful, well written, easy to navigate, and, with few exceptions, free. I have omitted information that, although important, can be found in more general cancer books, such as what steps you should take when first diagnosed.

In addition to the twenty- and thirtysomething cancer patient, this book is intended for friends, family, coworkers, spiritual leaders, and mental, medical, and allied healthcare practitioners. I hope these outsiders, through reading how we contort our bodies and minds to adapt to the young adult cancer experience, will gain insight into how to best tailor our care, diagnose us at earlier stages, respond to our needs, and befriend us at every phase of the disease.

It is a wretched and lonely feeling when our lives stump and bewilder those to whom we turn for comfort, solace, information, and support. It is utterly dumbfounding when our lives become so foreign to us that even we do not know how to best comfort ourselves. Through my conversations and research, I share the basic wisdom of practical experience and strive to show that there is no singular, quick-fix prescriptive for coping with cancer in your twenties and thirties. This learning is trial by fire.

1

Ramenomics

When Nora Lynch opened her mouth, an odd hybrid of British and Long Island accents flew out. As I hovered over a voice recorder for my first cancer conversation, this blind encounter with Nora held a palm-sweating edge strikingly similar to my first foray into the online dating world just two weeks earlier. Although I had previously carried on candid, one-on-one conversations about cancer with Seth—a lymphoma patient in San Francisco who became a close friend—our chats were absent a microphone and the expectation that our words would be immortalized in print. Nora was equally anxious because she had never encountered anyone her age who had cancer.

Nora had replied to my posting on the Washington, D.C., Craigslist. We exchanged a few e-mails and agreed that I would travel to the D.C. area. We met in a chaotic Metro parking lot in suburban

Virginia during rush hour. We each had an abbreviated list of physical identifiers so that we could recognize the other. Nora: a twenty-four-year-old woman, of medium height, with short black hair and pale skin. Me: a thirty-one-year-old woman, tall, with long brown hair. Nora looked Goth, clad in a black mesh shirt and black jeans despite the thick July humidity.

Seeking privacy from her two roommates, we parked ourselves on a cement-slab bench in a square in Old Town Alexandria. Loud buses hurtled past and kids screamed and splashed in a fountain as we took refuge in the story of the last nine months of her life. Despite my twinges of nervousness, I was confident about the parameters I had devised for these conversations. I had no prepared list of questions, I'd willingly share as much of my cancer experience with her as she wanted to know, and we needn't tell our stories in chronological order. We agreed that I could ask her anything, and she was free to skip over any answers and subjects that she wished not to talk about. Nora asked to use a pseudonym, out of fear that future employers could discriminate against her in the hiring process. She had just come from a doctor's appointment to have the site of her chemo port checked. I started our conversation by asking about her appointment, but she quickly dove back in time to the beginning of her saga. She spoke with biting humor and self-deprecation, mixed with intervals of steady, forthright contemplation.

"I was diagnosed with lymphoma nine months ago. During the whole nine months of cancer, I've had really great fantasies about finally being able to go to work. When I was diagnosed, I had just finished my graduate degree from the London School of Economics. I was so eager to be supporting myself and feeling like an adult at last. In college, everything was being done for me by someone else. My dorm rooms were found for me; my schedule was being set by someone else. I wanted to take care of myself for a change, but I suddenly entered this period of cancer, of not being able to do the most basic things for myself. It was like, Great, now that I've graduated college and am ready to become independent, I'll go back to infancy. I really feel like I was shot down by circumstances on the eve of becoming a financially independent adult.

"After I left London, I came back to Long Island, where I thought I was staying with my mother in her one-bedroom apartment for two weeks. I had a Long Island doctor look at this lump I'd found on my neck two weeks before, when I was finishing up my thesis in England. You know, when I got my positive biopsy report back from the doctor, I didn't even feel too upset. I kind of felt a sense of inevitability. 'Cause before I was diagnosed and telling friends and family that I might have cancer, they were all saying, 'No, no, I don't think you have it. I feel like you don't,' but my gut was saying something else. When I got the news, I thought, Okay, yeah, it figures, damn. I was a very casual smoker, maybe three cigarettes a week. I went outside and had a smoke and that's the last cigarette I've had. I didn't want to be one of those people standing outside a hospital with a drip in their chest smoking a cigarette. That's just too dark, even for me.

"My mom was at work when I got the news, and I knew she was going to freak out. Hearing her break down on the other end of the phone was probably the worst part of the entire cancer experience. She wanted to come home, but I preferred to be alone. My parents got divorced about two years ago. My dad. Oh God. Bless him, he can't help it. He's got obsessive-compulsive disorder and a whole host of other mental problems. When I called to tell him, he replied,

> "**People reading** this will think I'm crazy for smoking when I just got through brain cancer. I don't ever sleep and I'm going through withdrawal from being on high doses of pain medication for such a long period of time. I feel like I just need something to get me through but I do wish I could quit."
>
> —Krista Hale, 39

'Bummer. Seen that new Harry Potter movie?' I said no, and seriously, that was pretty much it. Once in a while he'd send me a postcard: 'So how's that cancer thing going, Nora?' It's like, Great, Dad, I'm having a great time. My grandparents tried to give us emotional and financial support as best they could. My sister is twenty-three. She came out from New York City quite a lot to check on us. But otherwise, it was just me and my mom. My mother had actually just been diagnosed with colon cancer two weeks beforehand."

As Nora spoke, I worked hard to bite my tongue, to not shout out, "What the hell are you talking about? You and your mom *both* had cancer, at the *same* time? How do you even begin to handle that?" I was shocked by how unfazed Nora seemed by the whole situation. Listening to her story, I so easily forgot what I have come to learn: that you play the cards you are dealt. You adapt. A life that appears freakish, bizarre, and extremely unlikely to the outside world can suddenly become normal to you because, really, there is no other choice but to move forward.

As Nora's situation spun in my head, I tasted some of what my friends experienced each time I dropped my little bombs of cancer news on them: "I have cancer." "My cancer has metastasized." "I need to repeat treatment again."

They either asked aloud or with a silent, quizzical look of wonderment the same question I now had for Nora: How do you *deal* with that? Sitting on this park bench, agape at Nora's situation, I realized that the inability to conceive of someone else's monumental distress is a luxury. There exists a thin threshold where concern for someone's well-being suddenly transforms into gawking. I caught myself at that threshold with Nora and decided that instead of asking how? why? what? I would do the best thing that anyone who knows someone with cancer can do: I simply listened.

"My mom and I were always really close, though we got a lot closer during our big cancer winter. We drove each other to chemo, spacing it so one would feel decent enough to do it for the other.

I wanted everything to be reciprocal like that, but I think she mostly took care of me because I was sicker. We lived under each other's feet that whole six months in a very small one-bedroom apartment. Occasionally, it would become a bit much, but we'd just snap at each other and get it over with. We're very similar, despite the fact that she's very religious and I'm not at all. We agreed that it sucks that we both had to have cancer, but I'm glad that we had it at the same time. We'd joke about it, asking if we could get two-for-one discounts.

"The financial implications of dealing with cancer are huge. As a student in Britain, I was treated like a regular citizen and got their national health insurance. If I had stayed in Britain, I would have been fine. A month before I came home, my mom had to drop me or my sister off her health insurance plan because her employer didn't want to carry two additional people. My sister has asthma, so my mom thought, 'Nora's healthy. Let's drop her.' When I was diagnosed, I had no insurance, no job, and about seven thousand dollars left over from my college fund.

"I footed the bill to see a doctor at Sloan Kettering; she seems to be the top lymphoma expert in the world. I got her consultation but couldn't afford to get treatment at Sloan because I didn't have any insurance. She set out a very aggressive chemo regimen. Some think of Hodgkin's lymphoma as the pussycat of cancer, a couple whaps of chemo and you're done. Non-Hodgkin's is a lot nastier because it moves faster and is harder to kill. Mine is somewhere between the two; it's a nastier, more ambitious version of Hodgkin's. Since my cancer is a weird variant, the doctor couldn't give me numbers on what my chances were.

"My original plan was pretty neat. I was going to apply for Medicaid and get treatment from my mom's oncologist, right in our town, but I didn't qualify for Medicaid because I had over two thousand dollars in savings. They instead

"**The idea** that there are 'good cancers to have' is a disgusting thought."

—*Brian Lobel, 23*

referred me to a state plan for people who are slightly less horribly poor, for people who have more than two thousand dollars in savings but earn less than seven hundred fifty dollars per month. The state insurance plan said, 'We pay for chemo, but we only cover certain drugs and yours are not on our list.' This is one week before I had to start chemo, and the doctor at Sloan had said I must start by X date; otherwise, the cancer may move so fast that my chances of surviving were going to decrease. It's like, I'm not calling to have my toenail removed, guys. This is kind of life or death. The state plan told me to apply for emergency Medicaid. By this time, I fit their criteria because in the three weeks since I originally applied, I spent more than five thousand dollars on hospital bills. Medicaid said they'd speed process me so I could start in a month or two. I needed to be halfway through chemo in two months.

"I just thought, Wow, I'm going to die because I have no money? I mean, I went to a succession of really, really good schools. I viewed myself, and people always told me, that I was a very promising person. And at the end of the day, the state didn't give a crap because I didn't have any income. They were kind of like, 'You can die, whatever.' That's when I really felt the 'Why me?'—not because of the cancer but because of the healthcare system. People aren't judging me as a person; they are only judging my financial situation.

"I couldn't wait for Medicaid to kick in, so instead of going to a private oncologist, I went up to a state hospital forty-five minutes away. I asked for a loan or financial aid. They were like, Fuck it, we'll just start treating you, sooner or later the money will come together. They didn't care. They were so used to people being in this financial situation. They said, 'We'll work out a payment plan. If it turns out you owe us thirty thousand dollars, then you can pay us over time.' In the end, the state hospital sent my bills to the state insurance plan that originally said it didn't cover any of my chemo drugs. The state insurance plan paid the hospital without even blinking. All that time,

I could have just gone to my mom's private doctor in our town, and instead I had to drive forty-five minutes to get to treatment at a state facility. They had, quote, just gotten it wrong.

"How do you deal with health insurance when the people who are administering it have no clue how it really works? The people on the phone at the state insurance office only have a high school education, and a lot of them hardly speak English. It is hard because these are very complex things they have to describe. I got so much wrong information, 'We don't cover this. Yes, we do. Maybe we don't.' When they tell you a doctor isn't in their plan, they are often working off information that is more than two years old. It's like, Get it right, God damn it, or find someone who knows what they're talking about because I can't sit on my ass and go, Well, maybe I'll get chemo or maybe I won't. To have to deal with that when you're very ill, even if you're completely healthy, it could drive you mental.

"At the end of chemo, my doctors didn't want to give me both the CAT and the PET scans because it was on the state's bill instead of private insurance. I thought, If I croak because they won't give me both scans, aren't they kind of wasting the money they've already invested in me? When I complained to my mom's oncologist, he said, 'Well, you're getting clean needles, aren't you? There are places in the world where

> "**I don't** make it common knowledge that I'm on disability, but I worked and this is my money coming back to me so I don't think I'm taking advantage of the system."
>
> —*Mary Ann Harvard, 24*

you wouldn't even get clean needles. You should be grateful.' After he left the room, I turned to the nurse and said, 'I can't believe he said this to me,' to which she replied, 'Well, it's *our* tax dollars.' I was like, Holy shit, do I have less of a right to live than people who are making ninety grand a year? I *am* begging, give me six months of life and I *will* have a job where I could pay for this myself.

"My doctors were very condescending to me. I don't know if it was because I was young or because I was a girl, or because they were burnt out and needed vacations, or a combination of all those things. I thought, Wait until I take over the world. They'll be the first ones up against the wall!"

Nora leaned forward into my tape recorder and spoke loudly and slowly: "Get jobs with benefits, everyone! Don't fuck around with not having insurance!" It was clear that Nora and I had both staggered through the wretched abyss of health-insurance hell. We were not members of that mythic tribe of young adults who are so often scapegoated by policy makers. According to the urban legend, a sizable chunk of our generation chooses to forgo insurance, cracks our heads open rock climbing, and allegedly makes the whole system go belly up. No, we were real creatures, typical twentysomethings, who got dropped from insurance while switching from college to the work world or from one job to another.

I had left my job three weeks prior to my own cancer diagnosis, and when I tried to make an appointment for a second opinion, I discovered that my employer had forgotten to submit my COBRA papers. I had cancer and no insurance. On the phone for weeks with my HMO, COBRA, and hospital administrators, I stretched the truth and fabricated enough red ink to reinstate my insurance and receive a second opinion from a prominent university teaching hospital. I successfully scheduled surgery and radiation treatment with top-notch doctors using fudged health insurance. Riddled with anxiety, I hoped that my house of cards would not come crashing down until I either obtained legitimate insurance or made it through treatment.

I needed a long list of questions answered about how to obtain legitimate, affordable insurance with my newly existing condition. Although the university hospital's facilities looked like a country club, with a reflecting pool in the lobby beside a grand piano, its social worker was useless. My own limited knowledge of applying for disability, which I had learned from a flyer, was greater than hers.

I dove into a long process of hard, desperate phone calling and found Nicola, a law student who took me on as a school project. We were the same age, and it put me at ease to talk about these overwhelming administrative issues with someone who was approach-able and did not scoff at my naiveté. She completed my paperwork when the side effects of my meds made my head spin too hard to concentrate, and spoke for me at my Social Security interview. She made the mysterious and intimidating healthcare system approach-able and surmountable. She helped me organize my medical records and legal documents and appealed for an eighteen-month exten-sion of my COBRA benefits and won. Nicola also discovered that the State of California owed me money for disability that I had not known I was entitled to. I cried the day that she brought me a $9,000 check, which without her help would have sat in the state's coffers instead of in my bank account. The money paid for my rent and groceries for an entire year.

I wanted to reach back into Nora's last nine months and hand her the gift of my health-law goddess. Although the system had ulti-mately provided her with chemotherapy, I knew that Nora would face a nerve-wracking challenge of finding insurance while she lived with a preexisting condition, received follow-up tests for years to come, and forged a new career path paved with temp jobs and bouts of unemployment. As I relayed my lengthy list of health insur-ance and financial resources to Nora, I realized that through years of hard work in trying to manage my own care, I had accumulated a wealth of knowledge. Transmitting this information to Nora helped me understand why I got so feisty when people assumed that as a cancer patient, my disease must have taught me about how precious and fulfilling life can be. I knew how precious life was before I got sick. What I had learned as a cancer patient was far more practical and lifesaving and much less glamorous: I learned how to navigate the labyrinth of health care in the United States.

The sun had set, and Nora and I left our park bench to roam the quaint storefronts of Old Town. Pausing in front of the Gap, I confessed that although I had loathed the girlie sport of clothes shopping for most of my life, I had become a closeted fashionista since my diagnosis. I was surprised to hear Nora agree.

"Yes, I also got really into clothes shopping during treatment. It felt like the most hopeful activity. Certainly, advertisers want you to shop all of the time with this level of intensity, but the only time I was that into it was when I was really fucked with cancer. I didn't have to buy anything. I loved just picturing myself in these new clothes. They made me think about what I'd be doing in the future, like going out and getting a job. It was so great imagining myself in a scenario other than chemo, where the only clothes I need are sweatpants, a sweatshirt, and a do-rag.

"I started losing my hair two days before Christmas. I wore this funky, straight black, shag kind of wig. Very Chrissy Hind. It lessened the blow of losing my hair because I just felt so fabulous wearing it, and I still wear it out, even though my hair has grown back. I've never been very girlie, but I became so much more so during treatment. I'd go into chemo with all of this Goth makeup on because it's the only kind I know how to do: black eye shadow, lipstick, nails. It helped me feel so much better.

"Treatment was depressing, but the most depressing part of cancer was being stuck on Long Island for nine months. Things never change there. After college, you feel like you've changed, your interests are different, and then you come back to this place where the last you remember you were seventeen, and there is no movie theater in town, there's nowhere that you can hang out. You just drink. It was uncool.

"I ended up working in the video store that I worked in before college. Because of chemo, I could only work one weekend every three weeks, but I needed to get out of the house and earn a little bit of money. People I'd run into at the video store who knew I went to undergrad and grad school in Europe would say, 'I didn't expect you'd be working in retail.' After a while, I started telling people about my cancer. I almost felt like less of a leper telling them that I have cancer than being like, 'Yeah, I'm stuck here on Long Island after graduate school for no reason at all.'

"It's weird deciding if I should tell people or not, but I needed to say it out loud, especially in the beginning, in order to believe it myself. When my coworkers and I were drunk in a bar comparing scars, I showed them my collar bone and was like, 'I have cancer. That is what this scar is from and I'm back on chemo in two weeks.' I was drunk enough it was funny to me but it was not funny to anyone else. There was a long silence, and people didn't know where to look. I was like, 'Hey, it's okay. I'm good with it. You should be, too.' Some people really had trouble talking to me afterwards; they'd look at me a little differently, with a strange shift of curiosity and sympathy, trying to see if my hair looked different, like I'd become a science experiment.

"I felt really alone at times. I met a lot of old women with cancer in the waiting rooms. They were nice, a little in awe of my age, and they all kind of babied me—even the nurses, too, because I was the youngest person they had ever treated. I really wish that there were people my age that I could relate to. Instead, my support group was *Buffy the Vampire Slayer* DVDs.

"I felt so depressed that I had spent so much time planning for my future and I wasn't even sure it was going to happen. I felt ill for so long that it just seemed like I was never going to be healthy again.

> "**I was so** nervous the first time I disclosed my cancer to a stranger. I took a coworker to lunch and I'm sure she thought I was going to ask her out. When I told her, she started crying hysterically. I was like, 'I can't tell anyone this news ever again.'"
>
> —*Matthew Zachary, 32*

I went through really bleak phases, but I didn't see a point in talking about it because I just thought it would bring other people down. I hated knowing that I made my friends uncomfortable, and I hated seeing them uncomfortable and listening to them denying that they were. I know it's contradictory, but even when people were saying, 'You'll probably be fine,' I'd feel kind of angry, like they weren't taking my cancer seriously, even though I also often didn't take it seriously in front of them either. I definitely thought about dying, and I still think about it all the time. Once cancer and the possibility of death are in your life, you see it everywhere. I manage to be mostly flippant about death. I tend to have a pretty morbid sense of humor, and I'm a worst-case-scenario person anyway. I've tried to talk to friends about dying, but they think I'm being over-dramatic, or it freaks them out too much to talk about it. I guess it's very different to think about yourself dying than it is for others to think about you dying. It must be so much harder to be the one left behind than to be the one who is leaving.

"I used to look at old people and think, Oh what a bummer to be that old and decrepit. Now I'm like, God, I hope I get that old. To be eighty and have the bus kneel for me, that would be so cool. I feel kind of confused and ripped off that I had to think about dying this early. During chemo, I felt like my life stopped before I'd just begun. At our age, death is what happens if you OD, or you drink and drive, or do something stupid that you could have prevented. It doesn't happen to you because of forces you can't control. I don't know. I'm sure that when I'm fifty, I'll be just as disoriented and horrified if my cancer comes

"**I like** the idea of an afterlife and I'm a sucker for near-death experience books. I really want to believe in these ideas but deep down I'm just too rational to think they're true."

—*Jill Woods, 38*

back. I suppose that's the arrogance of youth, to think you have to accept death at a certain age, but you never get to that stage, do you? Time will tell, I suppose.

"One of the things I was most proud of this entire time was that I did not waiver in my thinking that there is no afterlife. This belief stood the test of extreme freaked-outness. My mom relied very strongly on religion to get her through her treatment, and just about everyone I met who was getting chemo was very religious or going that way, it seemed, from the stress of the situation. My official line on it, before and now, is that you just can't know what, if anything, happens after we die, so you might as well spend your intellectual energy on things that you can know and can determine, things that you care about and can do something about. I think when you're done, you're done, and that's not necessarily a bad thing. I felt strength in that I didn't relapse into the religious faith that my mom pushed on me—thinking, This is happening for a reason, or, God will swoop in at the last minute to save your ass. I felt stronger that I continued to be able to not believe in religion, even though it could have been a comfort. When I went into remission, I had a couple of people say to me, 'Oh, God spared you.' I told them I think it's just that Satan hasn't got my corner office ready yet.

"It's been two months since I finished my treatments. I've moved from New York, and I'm working a temp job in D.C. I figure it is the best place to find a job in public policy. I no longer have any health insurance. I'm ineligible for Medicaid now because even though I only have eight hundred dollars in the bank, I have a job that's

> "**I get a twinge** of jealousy seeing my friends in the Peace Corps, backpacking through Europe, being nannies, and not worrying about health insurance. I'd like to be that innocent again."
>
> —Dana Merk, 24

going to pay me about thirty thousand dollars a year. Unfortunately, it doesn't have health insurance yet. I looked into purchasing private health insurance, but the premium was five times the normal rate, about fifteen hundred to two thousand a month. So I'm just going to pay the hundred and twenty dollars for my doctor visits out of pocket and basically hope my cancer doesn't come back. I still have to get blood work and scans done, and I don't know how I'm going to pay for that. Family loan time, big time. Honestly, it's such a grand scale—even if I eat nothing but ramen noodles for a month, I'll never be able to pay for it."

As Nora painted her financial reality, I thought about how young people have good reason to be cynical when we hear cancer described as an opportunity that makes us realize we should live for our dreams. For many of us, cancer is not necessarily an open door on the future, but rather an extremely large financial question mark upon which our big dreams hinge.

Nora and I had been sitting in my car in the crescent of her high-rise driveway for a half-hour. It felt like the end of a date, when you don't know what is supposed to happen next. We gave each other a hug and felt the awkwardness of parting after diving so quickly into our personal subterranean lives. She confessed that most of what she had told me, she had never talked about with anyone before. She thanked me deeply and sincerely. I watched as she walked through the lobby and disappeared into an elevator.

Two months later, I met up with a woman who had volunteered to transcribe Nora's interview; we'd also met on Craigslist. As she handed me the ninety-page transcript, I asked what struck her the most about listening to our recorded conversation. She said that Nora seemed nice and all, but it got really boring listening to someone talk about health insurance. I couldn't agree with her more. Talking about health insurance sucks. I smiled at her and said, "Welcome to our world, honey."

RESOURCES

Health Insurance and Financial Guidance

If obtaining stable health insurance were easy or affordable, there would not be more than 15 million uninsured young adults in the United States. They make up the fastest-growing population of uninsured Americans. Fight for your insurance and financial needs as if your life depended on it . . . because it does.

Quick Tips

- Read carefully. Insurance decisions may be the most important choices you make during your cancer care. Understand benefits, limitations, and qualifications and how different forms of financial relief impact one another before you apply for any healthcare plans, government aid, or other types of financial aid.

- Read the American Cancer Society's document "Health Insurance and Financial Assistance for the Cancer Patient" to learn the definitions of key health-insurance terminology. Download it from www.cancer.org or call 800-ACS-2345 (800-227-2345) for a free hard copy.

- Find an advocate or recruit a responsible friend or family member to help with paperwork and phone calls. Forewarn them of the persistence they will need to resolve these issues.

- Try to seek help from a social worker, either where you are receiving care or where you wish to receive care. If he or she is not helpful, then call a cancer or nonprofit healthcare organization that has a large department dedicated to insurance and financial advocacy, such as those listed on page 26.

- Be prepared for busy signals and lengthy waits or plan to leave a message when you call organizations that offer health-insurance guidance to cancer patients.

Get Guidance

The following organizations will provide health-insurance information and financial counseling:

Patient Advocate Foundation, www.patientadvocate.org, 800-532-5274. This foundation offers over-the-phone case-management services, educational materials, and live online chat options to assist you with insurance, employment, and debt-crisis issues.

American Cancer Society, www.cancer.org, 800-ACS-2345 (800-227-2345). Ask for a referral to a local ACS patient navigator, a social worker, or an over-the-phone health insurance information specialist. These counselors are available in many, but not all, states.

Leukemia and Lymphoma Society, www.lls.org, 800-955-4572. The information specialists in this society can help you understand basic insurance issues and can provide excellent resources and referrals.

CancerCare Assist, www.cancercare.org, 800-813-HOPE (4673). This organization's licensed social workers can help you understand what insurance and financial avenues may be available to you.

Call Uncle Sam

Social Security Disability and Medicaid, www.govbenefits.gov, 800-FED-INFO (800-333-4636). Medicaid and Social Security Disability are federal programs that are administered differently from state to state. Contact your state, county, town hall, and local health department to cover all of the bases. Applying for government and other benefits can be a lengthy and challenging process. Begin as soon as possible, and for greater success try to enlist the help of a legal advocate.

Lean on a Legal Advocate

The Cancer Legal Resource Center, www.disabilityrightslegalcenter .org, 866-999-DRLC (3752). This center offers national telephone assistance if you have questions about health insurance, financial assistance, consumer rights, and other legal issues pertaining to cancer, or if you need a referral to free legal assistance in your area.

Do a Web search for your state legal aid society or a legal clinic at a local law school to find one-on-one legal help with insurance and financial options.

Insurance and Money Matter Must-Reads

The American Cancer Society's booklet "In Treatment: Financial Guidance for Cancer Survivors and Their Families" is an essential guide that answers your financial and insurance questions. Download it at www.cancer.org or call 800-ACS-2345 (800-227-2345) for a free hard copy.

CancerCareAssist's fact sheet "Financial Help for People with Cancer" includes an excellent list of financial aid opportunities. You can download it from www.cancercare.org or call 800-813-HOPE (4673).

Georgetown University Health Policy Institute's state-by-state "Guide for Getting and Keeping Health Insurance" can be downloaded from www.healthinsuranceinfo.net.

Kaiser Family Foundation's "A Consumer Guide to Handling Disputes with Your Employer or Private Health Plan" is available at www.kff.org.

Extra Dough

CancerCare Financial Assistance, www.cancercare.org, 800-813-HOPE (4673). This organization offers funds for transit, home care, child care, and other needs. Its application process is quick and easy.

The Leukemia and Lymphoma Society, www.lls.org, 800-955-4572. This society provides up to $500 per year in patient financial aid to needy patients for transportation and specific drugs and procedures. It has a simple application process.

Net Wish, www.netwish.org. This organization will give you up to $500 in financial assistance from a mystery donor following an easy application process.

Road to Recovery, American Cancer Society, www.cancer.org, 800-ACS-2345 (800-227-2345). This program provides transportation to and from your medical treatments.

Patient Assistance, www.patientassistance.com, provides updated, easy-to-access information on more than 1,000 prescription drug assistance programs. Tools include online enrollment applications, automatic refill reminders, and discount programs for those who are ineligible for assistance programs.

Airfare assistance for cancer-related travel can be obtained from Air Compassion America, Corporate Angel Network, and Med Jet Assist. For more information, do a Web search for each organization.

Joe's House, www.joeshouse.org, 877-563-7468, is a national hospitality guide that lists discounted or free lodging for cancer-related travel.

Shed your shame and use your "cancer card" to ask for financial assistance, financial forgiveness, and scholarships. I have heard great success stories about everything from a doctor who forgave a $10,000 medical bill to patients' having their fees waived for yoga classes and gym memberships.

2

When G-d Things Happen to Sick People

Sheila Silver was not a warm and fuzzy cancer patient. She sounded matter of fact and skeptical when she phoned me three weeks prior to our get-together. Despite her icy demeanor, she was surprisingly persistent in her communication and agreed to meet for an in-person conversation on the condition that I protect her privacy by using a pseudonym for her in the book. Sheila was a thirty-one-year-old woman in treatment for breast cancer. I was excited to meet with her; how many opportunities would I have to talk about cancer with patients who didn't like to talk about it?

The ten o'clock news, fashion magazines, and fund-raising brochures brandish stories of breast cancer survivors who are social women seeking sisterhood, are prone to cathartic emoting, and are raring to give back to the cancer community. But what about the stories of patients who view the pink ribbon as a scarlet letter, who shudder at the thought of rehashing their cancer tales, and who approach their disease as a personal medical issue? Because of their desire for privacy, we hardly know that this kind of patient exists; we rarely hear their stories because they are not clamoring for microphones at rallies or sending their journals to publishing houses. I was honored to be invited into the home of such a patient.

Sheila and I met at a Metro stop in Arlington, the day after my conversation with Nora. We ordered to-go salads from a Starbucks across the street and walked to her studio apartment in a townhouse basement. A bed and a couch were the centerpieces of her home. The kitchen consisted of a dorm room–sized refrigerator stacked high with cereal boxes. Hand weights and plastic file crates brimming with paperwork were scattered about the floor.

I had grown a bit intimidated by Sheila before our recorded conversation began. On the walk to her apartment, she, an observant Conservative Jew, went off on a diatribe condemning interfaith marriage and other practices of Reform Jews—a group that includes me and my family. I had to continually remind myself that Sheila's blunt and opinionated manner was what compelled me to meet with her. We sat on her couch for four hours as she spoke with unrelenting seriousness and quick intelligence. What struck me most were her perspectives on privacy and her struggles relating to God. She asked that I spell God with the strict Judaic spelling: G-d.

"I don't go around blurting out my personal life to everybody that I meet or to acquaintances. Right now, cancer is such a huge part of my life, because I'm going through treatment, that I find it hard to have normal conversations without including the cancer. Therefore, I try to avoid having conversations at all. I either have to talk about cancer or not, but there's really no in between. I'm stuck in this awkward place because I just moved from Boston to D.C., I'm trying to set up a life for myself and meet new people, yet how do you meet new people when you're not being honest and truthful with them?

"I was diagnosed six months ago, when I first moved here. I had just filed for a divorce and was temporarily living with my sister when I discovered a lump in my breast. The initial tests revealed a great likelihood that I had cancer, but still I told nobody. Nobody. I kept this information all inside. I didn't want to scare anyone in my family if there was nothing to be worried about. When I finally got the news, it took me three days to muster up the courage to call my parents. Of course, my mom did not believe me at first because I hadn't even told her about the lump or the tests. She didn't even know what to say to me except, 'You are not in this alone. We are here for you and we'll figure this out together.' After that conversation, I felt better knowing that they knew, but I also felt worse because I was burdening them.

"My parents had connections to the Faulkner Hospital in Boston through my aunt. My mom and I met each other in Boston and consulted with a radiologist, a surgeon, and an oncologist at Dana Farber, who worked as a team to create a plan for me. I got a lot of special treatment because of the connection, so I was very, very fortunate. I chose to participate in a clinical trial to get chemo presurgery, to try shrinking the tumor so they could perform breast-preserving surgery. I was randomly assigned a drug that had terrible side effects. I flew to Boston every three weeks for it to be administered.

"I thought of moving back to Boston, but I just moved to D.C. and had only lived in my apartment for a couple of months. Dealing with the cancer was enough, and the thought of moving again was too much. Also, while my family knew about my cancer, I still had not told my friends. It took me a long time until I told anybody else. It was like this big secret for me. If I picked up and moved back to Boston, everybody would ask, 'Why are you moving back?' I'd have to deal with all these other people. My way of dealing with it was telling as few people as I possibly could and internalizing everything, because it was easier to me than talking about it. So, by staying put in D.C., it made it look like everything was fine.

"I eventually told a few of my friends once I started going back to Boston for treatments. It was really hard because my friends are all twenty-eight, twenty-nine, thirty, thirty-one. It's not like I'm in my fifties and I've had friends who have dealt with this. Nobody our age, at least in my circle of people, had experience with friends with cancer. I don't know how I would deal with a friend who has cancer, either.

"My friends say, 'Tell me what I can do. Let me know how I can help you.' I don't know what to say. Still to this day I can't express what I need from them because I don't know what I need. I don't know if I need support or if I need my space. I don't want people calling me every day or sending e-mail and cards because it's bad enough I think about it all the time anyway. I don't need phone calls every night asking, 'How are you feeling? How are you doing?' I don't need that, but I also don't want nothing. Sometimes my friends are better off not saying anything to me than saying the wrong thing. I need my friends to just be themselves, but they're not being themselves, they're being weird.

"Knowing what I need is just one of those things that I guess I'll eventually figure out. For the past six months I've been in treatment straight through, with little breaks in between. So maybe once all the major treatments are over, I'll be able to make more sense of it. It's been so intense going from one thing to the next.

"I don't tell people when I meet them that I have cancer. I'm afraid. I don't want to scare people off. Right now, it's easier for me

> "**Not everybody** with cancer wants to go to a support group. I never went because I just didn't like the idea of it. Everyone deals so differently, there is not just one way."
>
> —Mary Ann Harvard, 24

not to establish those friendships. Some people just put themselves out there more than other people, and I've always been a private person. I don't feel like going around advertising to every person that I meet that I have cancer. It's nobody's business. I'm hiding behind this huge scene, and that's something that I have to deal and cope with."

As Sheila spoke, I glanced down at my voice recorder. It wasn't recording. I asked her whether we could pause for a minute while I scrambled for back-up batteries and my emergency cassette recorder, but she continued talking. She told me about a friend who signed her up for a breast cancer walk-a-thon. Sheila didn't want to go but acquiesced because it meant a lot to her friend. She was irate when she found two different T-shirts in the registration package; Sheila's read SURVIVOR across the front. Sheila said that just because a woman has cancer doesn't mean she wants to parade around a park announcing it with a big sign on her chest.

I was relieved to hear the rarely spoken opinion of a woman who felt branded, not liberated, by the label of "survivor." I wondered how many other women felt similarly but wouldn't dare say so. Although I appreciate the distance our culture has traveled from treating cancer like a silent disease to instilling patients with a sense of vocal pride, I cringed when I attended conferences and read stories that made breast cancer seem like a celebrity status symbol. Sheila concluded that sometimes friends want to do things for you because it makes them feel better and not because it is actually what you want or need. I jammed new batteries into my recorder, and she continued talking.

> "With all the races, rallies, and walks people assume you want to be celebrated for having survived cancer. No! The last thing I want is people cheering me on because I had a disease that I didn't want, was miserable getting through, and wish I never had. That should not be my moment of fame."
>
> —*Jill Woods, 38*

"Dealing with the stress of cancer is enough, but the divorce at exactly the same time has been the worst nightmare ever. The divorce has taken so much out of me, and it's taken so much of my time and energy. Maybe it's a good thing; maybe it diverted some of my attention away from the cancer. It's hard to deal with both at the same time, and it raises more issues, just about future dating and starting a family. It complicates the whole thing tenfold. I feel bad for my parents because they want grandchildren. I don't know what I'm going to end up doing or if I'm going to have any choices.

"Life goes on, and when I do meet new people, make new relationships, cancer is going to come up, and I haven't thought about how I'm going to deal with that yet. Right now, I can't think that far ahead—I'm taking it day to day, just trying to get through these treatments. But at some point, cancer is part of my life, and cancer is going to be part of my history. It is going to be part of who I am, hopefully not such a big part as what it is right now. But I need to kind of get over that hurdle of talking about it and not being afraid of it.

"**Having cancer** is like having a C in a class but still getting an overall 3.5 GPA. You did fine and came out okay in the end but wish you didn't have the C on your transcript. You'll always have cancer in your history."

—*Brian Lobel, 23*

"It scares me to actually accept long-term goals and plans for myself. Would I even want to get married again, or am I going to be too afraid that I'm going to leave this person behind? I dreamed of being a magazine editor. Is that dream still something I should try to achieve? Or is my life going to be cut short, and it's a waste of time to try to get there because it's not going to end up panning out anyway? Part of me feels like I should take all the risks in the world because what do I have to lose? And the other part of me says, 'Stay back, don't take risks, because you have enough problems already.' I want to do both. Right now, I'm doing neither. I guess now I'm just stepping back and being very conservative.

"Spiritually, nothing links together for me anymore. I'm definitely struggling. I don't even know what I believe anymore about G-d. I was raised with a relationship to G-d, which I now question because I feel like, how could I put all of this trust in somebody or something and then be let down by it? Praying before was to thank. I never used to ask for anything. Now I pray for help. I am praying with a need, and I don't feel comfortable with that.

"I thought I had a grasp on my relationship to G-d, and I don't. None of it actually has order or makes sense. At this point, so many things for me are becoming questions. I guess now I'm just realizing that there are questions, which prior to cancer I didn't even recognize. I'm starting to sort out or deal with possible answers, which is something I never did.

"I don't know when, how, or if my belief is going to change back to the way it was, or if it's going to be different, or if I'm going to lose faith in G-d completely. And maybe there isn't a G-d. Or maybe there is a G-d, and it doesn't matter what you've ever done to show your belief or your faith, you're going to get screwed anyway, so it doesn't matter what you put in because you're going to get what you get. Are the events in our lives predetermined or random? Who knows? I can't make sense out of any of it.

"Not knowing how or if I'm actually going to be able to believe in G-d again is scary, it's unknown. I don't have the answers to anything. There are just too many things that are unclear and that are indefinable or unanswerable. My rabbi has been trying to have discussions with me, but I haven't really been reciprocating. He keeps writing me letters and trying to call

"**I was given**
a year to live but I cannot worry about dying because I think that God has my number and knows when it will be up."
—*Krista Hale, 39*

me, but I'm not ready. I still haven't figured out these answers for myself so how can I have a discussion or argue a point? I have to have some answers, and I feel like those need to come from within. He can guide me, lead me, and motivate me, but I feel like so much of it has to come from within. Until I'm at the point where I have some answers of my own, I don't really have anything to discuss with the rabbi.

> "I am spiritually moved at times but not by religion."
>
> —Brian Lobel, 23

"Growing up, G-d and Judaism were just part of who we were. It was forced upon us. I went to Jewish day school where these thoughts are instilled in your head, you don't really comprehend them or try to understand them or figure them out. They're just a given. I think all of this confusion and questioning that I'm going through right now will help me figure out more about myself and understand more about who I am or what I stand for. It's just part of introspection, I guess."

Sheila's reflections on faith reminded me of my own changed relationship to prayer and Judaism. Although I never believed in God, in my mid-twenties I began to attend Friday night Shabbat services as a way to feel connected to my mother and my grandmother. After I was diagnosed, I did not miss a week, even when I was unable to walk on my own and I arrived in sweatpants, with bandages adorning my throat. During the ten-minute silent mediation in the middle of the service, my heart leaped from my tightly wound body and connected to the ether, healing me from my week's hellacious cancer routine.

A few weeks prior to my meeting with Sheila, I received the first of many test results that showed possible cancer activity. It raised the question in my mind of whether radiation had been or would continue to be an effective treatment for me. While sitting at a picnic table in my backyard, I digested the news. I was afraid of dying, and I tried to connect to that sense of feeling something larger than myself, that big blanket of unnamable comfort I had found in prayer, but nothing was there. I cried a deep sob that had no sound, not because of the absence of whatever shred of connection I had felt to God or the Universe, but because I was relieved that the faith I had previously known suddenly evaporated. Such a feeling might cause panic for some people, but for me it instilled a sense of clarity. Pining for hope had become exhausting, and seeing things as they were was deeply relieving. It didn't mean that I no longer wanted to be well; it just meant that I would rely on earthly actions instead of spirituality in order to do so. My new paradigm felt realistic, sensible, and comforting to me. Since that day, I have thought of the universe only as a scientific location. I occasionally visit synagogue to carry on a sense of family tradition, and when bad cancer news smacks me in the face, I let it hurt until the sting dissolves. I listened as Sheila concluded our conversation.

"People say after treatment is all over, they feel kind of lost. Here you've had this regimen, all these steps to follow, all these appointments, and then suddenly it just drops off, and you have all this free time and you don't even know what to do with it. I'm not afraid of that happening. I'm looking forward to that happening, but people say that you can feel kind of unsettled about it all ending. Going from totally intense to nothing—I can see how that would be such a drastic contrast.

"I'm almost done with chemo, and then after chemo I get a two- or three-week break before radiation. I'll hopefully get it in the morning before work. It's going to be five days a week for seven weeks. Supposedly it's fairly tolerable; it's just really, really exhausting. Tired? No energy?

> "As soon as everybody starts putting family, friends, and money into perspective I'll put my health into perspective, but until then I'm still going to obsess about the little things."
>
> —Brian Lobel, 23

So you rest. I'll take tired any day over nauseous or other feelings. It's not going to be easy, but I'm just going to get through the chemo first.

"I'm hoping on Friday I'll get back to the gym. I've been walking and lifting my little weights, but I feel like I'm almost ready to go back to the gym. I love it when I can exercise. I just bought a bike at a yard sale. It's an awesome bike. I have a bike, but so much of my stuff is at my parents' house in Michigan. I don't have it here. It's just easier to live simply. My new apartment came furnished, so if I move, I'll just pack up and I'm on to the next place. At some point, I'll want to feel settled again and feel like a real person with a real place to live and real furniture, but for now, I'm kind of like a nomad."

It was dark outside when we finished talking, and Sheila drove me to the Metro station. There were no hugs good-bye or promises to stay in touch, as with Nora. I contacted Sheila a month later to ask her a few questions about the parts of our conversation that were lost during my technological meltdown. Sheila said she was very glad to have met me, but she didn't want to answer any more questions. She had met with me once, and that was all the talking she wanted to do.

RESOURCES

Spiritual Questions

Dissecting the purpose of hope, cursing the Maker, plunging into a vision quest with the Universe, finding peace with the unknown, pondering the afterlife, making meaning in the midst of chaos, rediscovering prayer, and concocting personal spiritual rituals—these are some of the spiritual challenges reported by young adults who discover they have cancer.

Whom do you turn to with these questions, curiosities, and conundrums? Where can you find comfort if you are living far from your family and the religious institution you were raised in? What do you do if you were questioning God or religion even before your cancer diagnosis? What can you do if your spirituality or religion no longer serves you during cancer or afterward?

What Is a Chaplain?

Erase from your mind the image of a chaplain as a prison pastor, a priest who only reads last rites, or Father Mulcahy from *MASH*. Chaplains are trained to give interfaith spiritual counseling and are available in most hospitals. The core of a chaplain's job is empathetic listening, helping a patient feel heard and understood. Chaplains are there to support a patient through fear, anger, and loneliness. Although you can request a chaplain of your faith to pray with you, chaplains serve patients of any faith or no faith, and it is unethical for them to proselytize or evangelize.

Throughout my cancer care, I had many meaningful experiences with chaplains, in which God was never even spoken about. A Baptist chaplain calmed my nerves in the pre-op room. A Jewish chaplain talked to me about my fears of death and dying. I'm an atheist and I think chaplains are the best-kept secret in the healthcare community, so chances are that almost anyone can find value in meeting with one.

Check off the box on your hospital admission form to have a chaplain visit your room, or ask a nurse or a doctor to page a chaplain who is on call, to visit you during day trips to the hospital. Many hospitals have a chaplain on call around the clock.

Seeking Spiritual Direction

Spiritual direction is a process that occurs as a one-on-one or group-counseling relationship in which you can explore spiritual experiences and receive support. Spiritual direction is offered for many different faith traditions. Some spiritual directors charge a fee and schedule regular appointments, much as a therapist does. To learn more about spiritual direction and to locate resources in your area, visit the Web site of Spiritual Directors International at www.sdiworld.org.

Mining Other Spiritual Resources

- You may have a favorite clergy member with whom you want to reconnect. Even if you have not spoken with this person in years, clergy are there to lend support when you need it most.

- If you are in school, look for a campus faith organization or locate a campus chaplain.

- Choose someone you know who is a good listener—a friend, a family member, or another cancer patient—who can give spiritual support simply by sharing in meaningful conversation.

- If you are seeking a contemplative practice other than prayer or in addition to it, explore meditation, spiritual journaling, spiritual drawing, making collages, singing, chanting, or taking a solo walk in nature or an unusual urban landscape that you don't normally visit.

The Best Spiritual Read during My Treatment

When Things Fall Apart: Heart Advice for Difficult Times, by Pema Chödrön (Boston: Shambhala Publications, 1997). You do not have to be a Buddhist to reap deep meaning from this Buddhist nun, whose writing cuts to the core of what it means to stare pain and suffering in the face and come out on the other side.

Critical Paperwork

The paperwork dotting Sheila's floor is a trademark of the cancer life. Cancer is often described as a physical, emotional, and spiritual

experience; for me, cancer was a physical, emotional, and administrative experience.

Organize Your Inner Admin

- Create a binder with contact info for all doctors, pharmacies,
  and medical records departments (fax numbers are extremely
  important). Keep a calendar for appointments, a log for
  medical phone calls and insurance phone calls, and a prescription log. Organize your insurance information, and save all
  receipts. You can download templates for these logs from www
  .cancerandcareers.org. On the home page, just click on "Charts
  & Checklists."

- If you are not a stellar organizer, simply keep a box where you
  dump every piece of medical information so that you can put
  your hands on it when you need it.

- The American Cancer Society's document "Health Insurance
  and Financial Assistance for the Cancer Patient" includes
  "Keeping Records of Insurance and Medical Care Costs." You
  can download it at www.cancer.org or call 800-ACS-2345 (800-
  227-2345) for a free hard copy.

- Make copies of your records as a backup and to give to
  doctors.

- Before leaving a doctor's appointment, ask for a copy of your
  pathology, lab, scan, or test reports to add to your file, to
  minimize your need to obtain these documents through the
  medical records department.

- When filling out a medical records release form, release as
  much information as possible—labs, slides, pathology—so you
  can have other institutions obtain as much of your medical
  information as you deem necessary.

Best-Ever Cancer Buy

A cheapo fax machine for sending medical release-of-information forms and records.

Advanced Directives

Advanced directives are documents that specify your end-of-life wishes. If pondering these documents freaks you out, lighten the blow by making a date with a healthy friend to do them together. This is a document that everyone should have, not only cancer patients.

Advanced directive is an umbrella term for two different documents: a living will and a healthcare power of attorney. A living will is a document that states your preferences for medical treatment at the end of your life. A healthcare power of attorney is a document that designates a particular person to make medical decisions on your behalf if you are unable to speak for yourself. For example, your living will may state that you do not wish to be kept alive on a ventilator for a prolonged period of time, and your healthcare power of attorney may designate your sibling as the person to enact these decisions on your behalf.

Moving out of state? Going to another state for your medical care? Be sure that you have an advanced directive for any state in which you receive care.

Download a state-specific legal advanced directive at www .caringinfo.org, or, for a more spiritual and holistic version of an advanced directive, visit www.fivewishes.org. Check to make sure that your state is on the list of locations where the Five Wishes version is a legal document.

Disability Papers

Paperwork associated with disability insurance is crucial since insurance may furnish you with income while you are sick. See Financial Guidance on page 25 for more information on Social

Security Disability and also see Employment Rights and Wrongs on page 98 for information on short- and long-term disability.

Wills and Life Insurance

Read *Be Prepared: The Complete Financial, Legal, and Practical Guide to Living with Cancer, HIV, and Other Life-Challenging Conditions* by David S. Landay (New York: St. Martin's Press, 2000), the most comprehensive and essential resource for information on wills, life insurance, and other legal and financial paperwork.

3

Single

My conversations with Nora and Sheila were a ripe confluence of intimacy and grit. They transformed the insidious cancer monologues inside my head into addictive dialogues. These conversations were like medicine, candy, or drugs, and I wanted more. Six weeks after meeting Nora and Sheila, I flew to San Francisco for an opinion about the suspicious nodes in my neck and scheduled a marathon itinerary of one-on-one cancer conversations: seven meetings with seven new patients in seven days. Although I was full of anticipation thinking of these new conversations, years of twisted cancer memories crept up from behind and lodged in my stomach. Most visitors stroll through San Francisco inhaling the smell of sourdough and gazing at the Golden Gate Bridge; to me, it would be a guided walking tour evoking memories of surgery, radiation treatment, and the heartache of serial dating with cancer.

Each neighborhood in San Francisco brought back stinging memories: the open MRI facility where they jammed my head into a plastic cage and scanned me for two hours to determine whether my cancer had spread to my sinuses; a doctor's office where, when I went ballistic on the incompetent staff, they threatened to have security remove me; a park bench overlooking the ocean where I sobbed my eyes dry after receiving bad test results; a tapas bar, a theater, a museum, a beach, and five apartment buildings where dead-end dates had led to kissing or sex but never commitment. When I turned onto Wafa'a Badriyeh's street, I discovered that her apartment was a block away from the house of an ex and four blocks from my hospital.

Like a loaded spring that burst the moment I walked in the door, Wafa'a was a quick distraction from my accumulating bad memories. Wearing yoga garb and sitting cross-legged on a scavenged couch, Wafa'a passionately dove into the story of coping with her lymphoma. As we spoke, her five roommates meandered in and out of the living room, nodding hello. Wafa'a was an open book, dishing out the intimate details of her dating life for all to hear. I was curious whether a woman as magnetic as Wafa'a—with her charismatic personality, shiny black hair, gorgeous face, and body that any woman would envy—was challenged by dating while she had cancer.

"Cancer makes you feel really alone, and you just want to be held and feel loved. Or maybe it is a coincidence, and I'd just really want those things right now even without cancer, and it's just part of being twenty-four. I want to matter to someone else. I want to feel like someone is thinking about me. Since being sick, I'm just looking for a bit of stability, and I think maybe having someone to love me is it. You can't control life so maybe you can just date and control that, but you can't control that either.

"When I was first diagnosed, I wondered if guys would be disgusted knowing there's this tumor inside of me. I felt tainted. Of course, I didn't want a guy to go away when he found out I had cancer, but I felt like it would be natural if he did. Who signs up for that? When you are in love, you will do anything for someone, but what about when you are just casually dating and you don't know the other person all that well? If I were just starting to date someone who was just diagnosed with cancer, would I worry about getting close and losing them later?

"I've been diagnosed three times in the past two years. I was in a four-year relationship the first time I was diagnosed. I eventually broke it off because he was more serious and settled than me, and I wanted my freedom and independence. Since then, I've been compulsively dating, so relationships have been mostly casual and fleeting. Because of cancer, I'm emotionally unavailable. I'm a wreck. I can't feel anything, I'm numb and in my own world.

"I was dating a guy for about six months when I got diagnosed the third time. We hung out the first week after my diagnosis, and then he pretty much disappeared without warning. If someone needs space, tell me. I'm totally understanding like that. When he got back in contact, he told me he just wanted to be friends. When we started, neither one of us was looking for a relationship, but you can't help it, you can still fall for somebody. I almost wonder sometimes if a broken heart felt worse than the cancer.

"I'm not ready for a relationship because I'm not stable, but on the other hand, I want to feel love. People really like me as a person and have such a great time with me, but they're not falling in love with me. And that's okay, but I want to feel special and I don't. There's something lonely at the end of the evening when there's no one out there that really misses you that you miss, too. I know there are guys out there that do feel that for me, but I want that mutual feeling. There's something so fulfilling about romantic love when someone who loves you looks into your eyes and all that cheesy stuff."

Wafa'a's transparency about her loneliness and desire to be loved was a relief to hear. It helped erase some of the shame I felt about the empty space in my bed and how I tried to fill it with a long string of men, whom I hoped would stay the night and just hold me. Although I quickly learned that my illness was a deal breaker for long-term relationships, dating remained my ultimate distraction. It replaced the anguish of cancer with the heartache of rejection.

> "**If I had** a message to the men of the world who have rejected women with cancer it would be fuck you! No. You're an idiot. No. You're just selfish. It's so pathetic—do these men not think that they could get sick some day too? It's just bad karma."
>
> —*Melissa Sorenson, 25*

I stopped dating a rabbi two weeks before my diagnosis, and although our ending was amicable, when he found out about my cancer, he never once called to ask how I was doing. I dated a painter for a year, who during my second dose of treatment sat by my side complaining about his need for solitude, as if time away from his easel was more painful than my cancer. I had recently broken up with a great man, who after a year of dating was still unable to say the word *cancer*. He referred to it as my "condition."

I failed each time I tried to stand in these men's shoes and empathize with their silence and apprehension toward me. I began to change my approach: I told men upfront about my cancer, received their excuses for why this could only be a casual relationship, bawled at home alone, then enjoyed a month or two of nice dinners and rolling in the hay with them before searching for the next guy. In my first two years of living with cancer, the number of men I slept with had more than doubled. Wafa'a continued talking about her track record with men.

"If you're a broke, unstable, unemotional musician, I'm dating you. When I date guys who are really together, they make me feel undone, unstable, so dating these other guys makes me feel more like the normal one.

"Some guys are also attracted to my messy life. One guy said, 'I feel like I'm a better man just knowing you.' I'm like, I don't make you a better man. I barely know you. Sometimes it is this romantic thing—Oh, she has cancer, she is so strong. They don't see the woman inside. They see 'survivor.' There is more to me than a strong survivor. I'm strong, but I'm not a rock. Sometimes I feel really tough and hard, and other times I feel like an open wound. I hadn't cried much the first couple years, but it all came out with the third diagnosis when this guy disappeared on me. I was a boiling pot for two years and I just exploded, and the steam is still coming out now 24/7.

"Being strong is not just about being inspirational or having your shit together. It's about being able to freak out, too, so long as you don't get stuck there. Being strong is admitting that you are vulnerable 'cause we don't want to believe that anything can affect us. I didn't. Are you kidding? I'm gonna go to school during cancer, I'm gonna be tough, nothing's going to affect me. You know what? It's affected me. I'm in shock right now. I'm freaking out. Maybe I'll start healing now that I'm actually able to be sad. I don't want this to go on forever because it's very draining, but in my weakness I feel stronger, in a weird way.

"When I get a cancer diagnosis, I feel sadness, frustration, anger, loneliness, and really violent, like I want to break something and freak out. Some people get anger out externally, but I take it out on myself. After the third diagnosis, I cut myself. I had a history of cutting myself when I was a teenager but had stopped mostly because I felt God was gonna punish me for it. I thought part of me getting cancer was God saying, 'You cut yourself, you tortured yourself, look what I can do, I can be a lot harder.' As I kept getting sicker with cancer, I got out the razor and I cut myself again. I felt stupid, like, 'I'm twenty-four years old, why am I cutting myself? I'm too old for this.' One night in the shower I was just freaking out and almost contemplating killing myself. I told my dad, 'Here's the razor, here's everything, hide it, take it away.' I haven't cut myself since then. I have scars that I gave myself and I have scars that cancer gave me. I look at my body and think, What a mess.

"I don't feel sorry for myself or angry at the world, but the wear and tear of cancer catches up with you. Recently, the only deep relationship I've had was the guy who disappeared. All of my closest friends have moved to other countries, other states, or are traveling. Nobody around me now has known me more than a year, it seems. All my rocks, all my stability, nobody was around, and I think that's why I freaked out; I didn't have the cushion around my heart that was always there before.

"Friends come and go. Social groups change. I don't trust anything in my life that's here today will be here tomorrow. The lack of stability is so tiring, but you embrace this insanity 'cause it's all you can do. You don't want to hate it, you don't want to be afraid of it 'cause it's you. This chaotic life is me and that's all I have, and so you kind of find ways to love it. But it's hard to love 'cause it doesn't always love you back.

"Doctors tell you to look for signs of recurrence. I'm walking a thin line between being conscious of my health and feeling like a hypochondriac freak."

—Dana Merk, 24

"With cancer, there is a residue of fear and distress and pain that doesn't go away even after treatment is over. I get this anxiety and fear where I can't be alone, so partying is my drug. Even though I don't do drugs, the dancing and the excitement of meeting new people, the whole scene, is the biggest high. Thursday through Sunday, and sometimes Monday or Tuesday, I'm out on the scene, dancing until 5 A.M. I may only get three hours of sleep before I go to work, but I'm having a good time. When I'm not out, I get depressed, I feel lonely, I come down. All these things are an escape, a distraction. If I was really happy, I could sit at home and watch a movie and feel good about that because I'd be happy within myself. Instead, I feel like, What if I watch TV and die tomorrow, was that wasted time? It's a whole different world at this age, being out there and dating. At eighty, I might not be so down if I'm at home having to watch TV, but at twenty-two I'm not ready to be sick and in a hospital for months at a time. I'm not ready to die. In the club scene, you just forget that you're sick and you can just dance and talk and flirt.

"A friend visited from Germany, and we went to a club. He kept asking, 'How are you feeling?' He was always trying to go inward, and he wouldn't let me escape. It was actually the best thing for me. I visited him in Germany and went to museums and talked and had real discussions about my fear. He taught yoga, and I went to his class once. People were always telling me to do meditation, do yoga, and I'm like, 'No, I don't want to think. I don't want to be real. I'm trying to forget. Don't ask me to stop running.' I started crying in the middle of class 'cause we were pushing our bodies so much, and I felt like my body is this worthless piece of crap. I had mono when I was twelve. I've had bronchitis. I've got all these scars. I've had cancer. I really feel like a defective unit on the assembly line, like God messed up. I walk around in this shell that's breaking down, and it's supposed to be my heart and my soul that makes this all okay, but that's being broken down, too. Everyone's like, 'You have to make yourself happy,' and I don't know how to do that.

"**If you are** older, I hate to say it but your boobs are already sagging. Having my body mutilated as a younger person has to be harder because I'm supposed to look in the prime of my life."

—*Jill Woods, 38*

It takes men, parties, my calendar being filled to give me the illusion of happiness, but at the end of the day I still feel alone.

"I live in six-month blocks from scan to scan, so I can't make plans more than six months at a time. I would love to be able to think five years out from now, but I can't. It's really tiring seeing the potential for more sickness coming. Everyone says, 'Well, you could die tomorrow, you could get hit by a bus,' and I know that. But you don't see the bus coming, you don't spend today thinking about it 'cause getting hit by a bus is random. When you have cancer, you're so aware of your life, your mortality. I want to live my life, but I feel like I'm testing fate or jinxing myself if I make plans for having a family, a career, and they'll be taken away from me. I can't even buy plane tickets a year in advance. I live day to day so I don't get disappointed.

"Next month I'll be moving apartments for the third time in three months. I've been subletting. I can't make a permanent move yet 'cause I don't know how my CT scans are gonna come out. With cancer, you almost feel like you don't want to stay anywhere too long 'cause it can be taken away from you. So as long as you get up and leave, you're the one who's taking control of your life. I'm making things happen instead of letting them happen to me. I've learned to deal with this short-term mentality. Stability and long term don't feel normal to me anymore. Having something for one month or two months feels safer. Before cancer, I would be able to sign a six-month lease or sign up for a year at the gym, but now everything I do is month to month.

"Three months ago, I moved out of my family's home for the first time ever, and it's exciting having independence, my own place, my freedom. Cancer would be less scary if I could still be independent. I hate the idea that I am helpless and have to rely on family to take care of me. I don't want to have to need them.

"My parents are very much there for me emotionally, of course, but for a while they did drive me nuts. When I was living at home during treatments, I had to make my bedroom a sanctuary. I spent all my time in there with my books and my music. I'd light candles and listen to Nina Simone or Portishead and write, or read *The Unbearable Lightness of Being*.

"My parents were so smothering, controlling my eating habits, medication, how much I slept, what I was wearing, if I was keeping warm. It made me feel sick all the time. I know it was because they love me so much, and they didn't know what to do. Parents think they're gonna be the ones to get sick first, so when their kid gets sick first, they're not expecting that, and it feels unacceptable. They want to take away the cancer and make everything okay, and they can't.

"My parents always try to fix everything, but sometimes I just need to vent. They try to encourage me by telling me all the time that others have gone through this and are fine. I feel like they don't get it. I'm not asking them to make me feel better; I just want them to listen. There are no answers, no solutions, just love me, be there for me, let me vent. When my dad tells me to be positive, I think, You have no idea what it is like to have cancer for two years. Don't I deserve to cry once in a while? I need to let it out. My initial reaction is to get angry at him, but I do know that deep down he is really scared that I might not be okay. Who suffers more, the people with cancer or the people around them watching them go through it and they can't do anything?

> "**I fought** with my husband over a fucking Krispy Kreme. I snuck one from the kitchen when I wasn't supposed to eat anything from the outside world because of bacteria. I cried and cried and was like, 'Don't touch me. I hate you guys all treating me like a child.'"
> —*Amilca Mouton-Fuentes, 26*

"My mom never wants to hear me say anything bad when I'm freaking out in between my scans, as if my worrying will give me bad test results. If there's a tumor in me, I can be as positive as I want, but it's still gonna be there when I take the scan. I don't want to pretend. It's so much worse to be a hundred percent positive and then get slapped in the face. For me, it's easier to expect the worst. It's not as much of a letdown.

"I have family in Lebanon and in Jordan, and it is interesting to see who among them wanted the details instead of just pretending it's not there. If you have a stomachache in Lebanon, everybody's trying to help you and talk to you about it. If you have cancer in Lebanon, no one even brings it up. They'll talk your ear off and diagnose you over the common cold, but when you talk about death or cancer, it's kind of taboo. They just pray, pray, pray for you on their own and give you big hugs. I know they care so much, but they don't ask questions or talk to me about it. Whereas in Jordan, when I was sick, they really asked me questions. They were interested in the details, in understanding my illness, in e-mailing and following up. When you have cancer, you see who really—I don't want to say who loves you more, because I know my family in Lebanon loves me just as much, maybe more, but you see who's not afraid to get real with you.

"Cancer has made me so real. I feel like I'm so raw, like there's no time for bullshit. Life is short, and I don't want to waste a minute of it trying to be cool or holding my shit together. Cancer has kind of given me an extra backbone. I've become very outspoken. I'm just not as nice as I used to be, like if a guy's bothering me at a club, I tell him. If a friend's asking too much, I'm just like, 'I can't

> "**I was overwhelmed**
> by crescendos of emotions and I cried. I'd go to my bedroom, close the door, put on my headphones, and just lay there for a couple of hours and deal with it."
>
> —Rick Gribenas, 28

> "**Cancer made**
> me want something better for myself than the men I had been dating."
>
> —Melissa Sorenson, 25

deal with this. I have enough in my life.' If I care about someone, I don't want to play games. It's tiring.

"I really started to accept death and dying more during my last treatment. It started feeling like maybe I shouldn't do treatment. Maybe I should just quit my job and travel and enjoy myself. I started to prepare myself for it more mentally. What scared me more than dying was what happens when I start to get sick and feel suffering and pain. Cancer can be a horrible way to go, I think. I believe in God, but I have no clue what happens when you die. I don't have faith in heaven or hell, so I don't have the idea of heaven to keep me safe. I have thought about it, and I don't know. Maybe it is just silence. That would be a relief.

"If I die tomorrow, I think I've done a lot. I've traveled all over the world. I've been in love. I've had really good friends. I've lived on my own. Is it okay to go because I have done so much? I try to find ways to make myself feel better about dying. At times, it was easier for me to accept death than to fight it. The scans, biopsies, paperwork, chemo, radiation, appointments, I'm just so tired of it, and at one point I thought if this is just going to be my life, maybe I don't want to be alive. I feel like an old, old soul, and cancer aged me a lot, too.

"Right now, I just tell myself what I would tell anyone who just got diagnosed: It's just one day at a time. Remember to breathe. Be a little selfish and don't feel guilty. Tell people how you feel and be open. Remember to tell people that you love them. Don't play games, don't be fake, don't try to be tough all the time. If you need denial right now to get through, do it. If you need to cry and feel it every day, do that, too. You're not alone, no matter how alone you feel, and you will feel alone, 'cause you feel like you're the only one going through it. And we are, because we're all different in our own way. But there are people out there that can kind of understand, and when you're ready, they'll be there for you."

Forget therapy, social workers, and self-help books. Nothing could beat the cancer credo that had just flown out of Wafa'a's mouth.

Talking with Wafa'a was engrossing, yet after six hours of whirl-wind conversation I was exhausted. We hugged good-bye, and I walked toward the BART station. Like Wafa'a, I was always try-ing to find the party and hated to be alone. But after our conversa-tion, instead of making plans with one of ten San Francisco friends, I headed back to the apartment of my friends Josh and Louesa, where I was staying. They were out for the evening, and I indulged in the rare experience of spending the night alone reading magazines and playing with their hound dogs. Wafa'a settled into my system like a homeopathic antidote, a concentrated dose of fear and anxiety that for one evening mellowed my own racing and intense mind.

RESOURCES

Dating

I always thought that cancer and sex was fend-for-yourself, trial-and-error territory until I spoke with Sage Bolte, ABD, LCSW, OSWC, the Dr. Sue of the young adult cancer world. An oncology counselor for Life with Cancer, Sage educated me on the nitty-gritty details of cancer dating, sex, and the body image issues that we all think about but rarely discuss out loud.

When and How to Reveal Your Cancer

On the fourth date. Why reveal your cancer on the first or second date to someone you don't know, don't trust, and may not see again? By the fourth date you may know if you want to continue seeing the other person. If your cancer turns out to be a deal breaker, hopefully you have not gotten too attached to him or her.

There are exceptions to the fourth-date rule: If your cancer is visible, you may prefer to address it up front. Also, if you have a tell-all personality, it may feel right to disclose your cancer on the first date. Don't wait too long though; if you reveal the truth two or three months into dating, the other person might feel you have been dishonest or withholding information.

Sound empowered and informed. Know your disease and your fertility risks so you can answer questions the other person may have. The more knowledgeable you are, the more you will feel in control of the situation.

Know how much to say. Don't spill your entire cancer story at once. Too much information can be overwhelming. Remember, cancer is one part of your life story; don't let it overshadow the goals, aspirations, career interests, and other life stories you would normally share.

Practice makes perfect. Practice out loud with a friend what you will say on a date. The more comfortable and casual you are with your "script," the more it will sound like another part of your larger life story.

In case of rejection. The bottom line is, if you were rejected by someone because you have cancer, do you really want to be with that person anyway? Now, does that question make you feel better? Didn't think so. Bash the one who rejected you in a support group or with friends. Get it out of your system so you are ready to move on and find a stellar human being who is thrilled about you and what you bring to his or her life.

Cancer Sex Ed

Common Mechanical and Emotional Challenges

Don't feel like a freak. The following challenges are common among many young adults with cancer: decreased libido during and after treatment; difficulty maintaining a firm erection; vaginal atrophy and stenosis (a narrowing of the vagina), which can be a side effect of pelvic radiation or a graft-versus-host-disease, or be caused by a break in sexual activity; and vaginal dryness from treatment or menopause. Sex may be emotionally challenging due to stress, anxiety, or depression and physically challenging due to scarring, loss of body parts, or maneuvering prosthetics or apparati like a port or colostomy pouch.

Newcomers and Those Returning from Vacation

If you were not sexually active prior to cancer or have taken a long vacation from sex, it can be difficult to know which sensations are normal and which ones should lead you to seek the advice of a doctor or gynecologist.

Talk to your doctor if you experience any of the following symptoms: for guys, inability to have or maintain an erection, consistent or persistent early ejaculation, or bleeding or pain from anal sex; for women, persistent internal or external vaginal dryness, persistent or consistent pain or burning in your vagina, or the feeling of tearing.

Sex Talk with Your Doc

Talk to your doctor before engaging in sexual activity to make sure it is not a contraindication with your treatment or surgery. Even if you are not sexually active at the time of your cancer care, it is important to talk to your doctor about the long-term sexual implications of your treatment. Doctors should raise these issues with you but most do not. Be assertive and proactive. No matter how uncomfortable you may be, be sure to raise your sexual questions. If your doctor is dismissive, ask to consult with a doctor who is knowledgeable about sexual issues and willing to discuss them and brainstorm preventative care measures.

Rethink Your Sexual Self

You have a sexual self that exists independently of the sexual act itself. It has been present since you were a kid, and having cancer does not take that part of you away.

With cancer, sex can become more of a mental than a physical experience; for example you might feel interested in another person but not get hot and wet. You should never force your body to do something you don't want to do, but if your goal is to become sexually intimate, you will need to work creatively with your mind to coax your body into the mood.

Spontaneity is an expectation for young adults, but with lowered libido and menopause you cannot always dive into the sack and make it happen. Forcing yourself to have sex often results in frustration and defeat. Instead, focus more on foreplay, structure, and planning. With sexual response problems, removing spontaneity is actually helpful. Is this completely unromantic? On one hand yes, and it sucks as do many other facets of cancer. On the other hand, it may open you up to romantic or kinky options you would never have otherwise tried.

Crack Out the Calendar

Choose one or two days of the week to be sexual with yourself or a partner—for example, every Tuesday and Friday. Use the few days before your designated days to mentally prepare, so your mind has a greater chance of getting your body to cooperate. Think of it as extra long foreplay: offer yourself positive thoughts; remember the enjoyable outcome of the last time you were intimate with your partner or yourself, regardless of how much work it took to get there; do things that make you feel extra beautiful; leave love notes; rent a romantic movie; find ways to tease each other.

Beyond In and Out

Here is a secret most people our age don't know: you can have extremely gratifying, sexy, hot, kinky, loving, romantic, and intimate relationships by touching, cuddling, kissing, and other kinds of sex that do not include penetration. *The Guide to Getting It On* by Paul Joannides (Oregon: Goofy Foot Press, 2007) is a thorough, funny, and sensitive sex guide, which normalizes positions, fantasy, masturbation, and sex techniques that will make penetration seem passé. Enjoy reading it as a couple or alone. Note that illustrations and language are quite graphic.

Know Your Body and Share What You've Learned

Spend time alone in the bath or in bed exploring your body to find what positions are comfortable, if penetration is painful or pleasurable and how deep you can handle it, and what body parts you do or do not want touched. Knowing your body and clearly communicating your needs to your partner will decrease anxiety for both of you.

This Is How We Do It

"Sexuality for Women and Their Partners" and "Sexuality for Men and Their Partners" are available from the American Cancer Society. Download them at www.cancer.org or call 800-ACS-2345 (800-227-2345) for free hard copies. These booklets offer great technical advice for dealing with sexual problems including how to stay wet, achieve the big O, work out your sex muscles, avoid pain, and manage erection issues. (Note: While most information can be adapted to all sexual orientations, it is presented from a very heterosexual perspective.)

Check out Planet Cancer's Dating, Relationships, and Sexuality forum for young adult cancer discussions ranging from masturbating in the hospital to how to hide your feeding tube with a corset during sex. Visit www.myplanet.planetcancer.org and click on "Forums," then "Dating, Relationships, and Sexuality."

Go Sex Shopping

Prolonging creams, heighteners, lubricants, vibrators, dildos, vaginal dilators—continue your sex education by perusing these products online either alone or with a partner. If your cancer is estrogen or progesterone sensitive, check with your doctor before using some of these products.

Pure Romance is a softer, less graphic online sex shop with a general shopping section plus a product line designed especially for cancer patients. Visit www.pureromance.com, select "Programs" and then "Sensuality, Sexuality, Survival."

Visit www.goodvibes.com to learn creative sex solutions by browsing their products that range from gentle to hard core.

Best-Ever Sex and Cancer Story

In her essay "Sex and the Sickbed," the writer Jennifer Glaser reveals the raw and sensual experience of dating someone with cancer. Read the piece in *Twentysomething Essays by Twentysomething Writers* (New York: Random House, 2006) or online in the *New York Times* archives, at nytimes.com; search "Jennifer Glaser."

Body Image

Body image issues are not a picnic at any age, but they are even more challenging in your twenties and thirties when people are more focused on superficial appearances. How you deal with body image issues such as hair loss, sudden weight loss or gain, saggy skin, stretch marks, scars, amputation, being a women with a missing breast, or being a guy with chest muscles that have not resettled to their precancer state depends on the intensity and severity of your personal experience.

If you are having an extremely rough time adapting to body changes, then creating a positive body image is not going to happen overnight; the process of grieving and redefining your self-image could take close to a year. The first step is to recognize you are having a hard time and then find someone you trust to talk to: a close friend, nurse, social worker, a support group. If you continue to feel horrified by the way you look, then it is time to speak with a therapist.

If recreating your body image feels challenging but manageable without therapy, here are some ways to work toward a healthier, more loving self-image. Again, there is no quick fix magic bullet here, but simply taking steps to transform your thoughts from harmful self-messages into positive ones can be very empowering.

The Mirror

For two weeks, look in the mirror when you wake up and instead of thinking negative thoughts feed yourself positive ones, even if you feel like you are bullshitting yourself. After two weeks, notice if there are any differences. Have positive thoughts about your body become more automatic?

Scars

Go out of your comfort zone. Find a very close friend of the sex from which you choose your sexual partners and show him or her your scar. Engage your friend in a conversation: Does my scar scare you? What do you think about it? Often our self-perceptions are worse than other people's perceptions of us.

Capitalize on the Good

Cancer has not changed everything about your body. Notice and dwell on the parts of you that you still find attractive, such as your smile, your eyes, the sound of your voice.

You're Just Projecting

When you project outwardly what you feel inwardly, it only exacerbates what you feel inwardly. If you used to wear makeup but stopped, try wearing it again. If you are only wearing ragged sweatpants and

T-shirts, find clothing that is comfortable, enhances your beauty, and makes you feel sexier. Use these resources for help:

Facing the Mirror with Cancer: A Guide to Using Makeup to Make a Difference. This makeup book for men and women with cancer, by Lori Orvitz, includes great tips on covering scars with makeup. Purchase it online at www.facingthemirror.org or order it from a bookstore.

Look Good Feel Better for Men and Women, www.lookgoodfeelbetter .org, 800-395-LOOK (800-395-5665), provides information for men and women on hair care, head coverings, skin care, and makeup. Women can also locate an in-person support group or schedule a free makeover consultation and receive a free beauty kit. If in-person programs are not available in your area, ask to receive the free video *Just for You: A Step-by-Step Guide to Help You Look Good Feel Better during Cancer Treatment.*

Skin Deep

An online safety guide for cosmetics and personal care products, Skin Deep, www.cosmeticdatabase.com, allows you to search for makeup and products that are free of known carcinogens.

Free Wigs and Other Beauty Items

American Cancer Society, www.cancer.org, 1-800-ACS-2345 (800-227-2345). Contact ACS to see whether your local office participates in a free wig program, can give referrals to other free wig programs in your area, or offers a $75 wig voucher.

Shop Well with You

Shop Well with You, www.shopwellwithyou.org, is a body-image resource for women with cancer. It offers "what to wear" suggestions, fabric guides, a clothing and accessories directory, and tips on how to use everyday clothing to feel comfortable and confident, inside and out.

Relationships

Among young adult patients cancer affects relationships in different, and often more challenging ways compared to older cancer patients. Sexual complications may take center stage for the twentysomething couple, for whom sex two to three times a week is the norm, whereas sex might be an afterthought for a seventysomething couple, for whom sex on average occurs less than twice a month. Many of our relationships are fresh and new, and we are just starting to learn how our partners respond to major life stress. And, with a national average divorce age of thirty years old, many of our partnerships are prime targets for hardship even before cancer strikes.

Whether your relationship is rock solid or on the rocks, cancer impacts every intimate partnership. Common challenges include diminished alone time, feeling guilty, wanting to protect each other from difficult emotions and fears of mortality, derailing goals and life plans, differing approaches to healthcare decisions, coping with denial and waves of emotions on different time cycles, different visions about how to return to life after treatment, financial challenges, interruption of your regular activities as a couple, and shifts in homemaking, bread-winning, caregiving, and childcare responsibilities. The following are basic relationship to-do's for any cancer couple.

Talk it out. Communication is essential to any good relationship. Even couples who normally excel at communication can be challenged by talking about the extremely difficult issues that cancer presents. Take time regularly to talk with each other openly about your fears, frustrations, and other feelings. Counseling can assist in this process and is a great tool to use not only when a problem exists, but to prevent problems from arising. See Emotional Support on page 146 to learn how to find a therapist.

Time away. During cancer care, it is easy to become glued to your partner both out of emotional need and in order to address your neverending medical and practical to-do lists. The healthiest relationships include some time away from each other. Plan for some time spent apart, even if only for a few hours per week.

Turn to a friend. Make sure you and your partner each have a close confidant with whom you can vent about the stresses of cancer and how it is affecting your relationship. Young adult cancer support groups and chat rooms are also great places to discuss relationship challenges and learn from others who are coping with similar situations.

Know You Are Not Alone

Divorce is a taboo topic in the cancer world, where stories of supportive husbands and wives are plentiful. If your relationship is not surviving cancer, know that you are not alone. In fact, the divorce rate for terminal cancer patients is higher than the national average. Learn more about cancer and divorce by listening to or reading a transcript of the American Cancer Society's Cancer Survivors Network online talk show on divorce. Visit www.acscsn.org. Select "Talk Shows and Stories" from the menu on the left. Then click on "Talk Shows," and scroll down to select "Divorce."

4

Human Spectacles

The next day while Josh and Louesa were at work, Amilca Mouton-Fuentes and I lounged on their sun-drenched couch talking for four hours. This couch was the cornerstone of my Bay Area cancer life. The first time I ever spoke the words "I have cancer" was while sitting on this couch two years earlier with Josh. His response: "Cancer. That sucks, but I'm not surprised. It's so Kairol— very dramatic." Even cancer did not faze Josh's biting sarcasm, and I soon came to prize the rarity of a response to my cancer that contained no posturing, pity, or fear.

In the midst of the touchy-feely Bay Area, Josh and Louesa's home was a no-bullshit bastion of grounded reality. No psychobabble hand-holding, no apologies, they wanted to be with me when I was at my worst, aching over cancer and kvetching about being single. Living alone with cancer in a city where I had little family, I felt at home in Josh and Louesa's small apartment. They unfolded a sofa bed (a mere four feet away from their own bed), forsaking their privacy on my behalf, night after night. Perhaps it sounds seedy, but when I was with them, I felt like I was in a relationship. I had a key to their house, and they were the ones whom I could come home to. They were there for me, no matter what.

Invincibility looks good on your cancer résumé; it gets you what you want in doctors' offices, makes you more charming at dinner parties, and increases your overall attractiveness to men who are slightly freaked out about the possibility of your dying on them. But at its core, invincibility exhausted me. At Josh and Louesa's, I never had to feign strength, resolution, or a positive attitude. Josh didn't just give me permission to let down the taxing guard of invincibility; he practically demanded it, with his constant reminders that my glass just might be half empty. Josh always saw the worst-case scenario in any situation, a finely honed skill only matched by that of my father.

Josh's perpetual, wry reminders that my life kind of sucked felt refreshing because it was the truth. I quickly tired of being the target of other people's unfounded optimism about my cancer: "You'll be fine, I'm sure." (How do you know that?) "You'll pull through." (Maybe, but at what cost to my body and my mind?) When it comes to cancer, this culture certainly hopes for the best, but we never prepare for the worst. At Josh and Louesa's, being my worst was expected and encouraged, and it allowed for both piercing humor and real sadness to emerge.

Sitting on their couch with Amilca was apropos; she was the first cancer patient I spoke with who let herself bawl while she was talking. Amilca's tears, snot, and Kleenex didn't make her fragile; in fact, they made her seem tougher. Out of everyone I met, she most reminded me that being badass and vulnerable were not mutually exclusive. This large woman with a pink Indian-print shirt, big hoop earrings, and peach-fuzz hair sat across from me on the couch and showed me what it means to live with the stench of cancer. Her fear was not tinged with anxiety, but rather an eyes-wide-open look at what had happened to her twenty-six-year-old body and what her future might hold.

"Way before I was diagnosed, I knew I was being called to do something. I kept saying, 'I'm about to step over a threshold, but I don't know what it is.' When my son was born fifteen months ago, I thought the universe was saying motherhood was going to be my great calling. I love my son, but I couldn't see being up to my neck in poopy diapers as being my great meditation. I'd rather keep looking for a while. I don't think the universe was preparing me for motherhood. It was preparing me to sit down, play some cards with death, and see who wins.

"Facing death is the most painful thing I've had to go through, but it is the greatest gift I have ever been given. I used to think that my son was the greatest gift. Or that my husband, Paul, was the greatest gift. I do think they are great, but I think that facing my death through cancer has taught me how to love them in a way that I never would have loved them before. So even if my time here is shorter, I'm loving them in the right way. I see death as a friend. It makes me stronger.

"Cancer awakened me to how I deny my body's needs. I must have known I was really, really ill. I got intense migraines, my vision changed, I had flus that I couldn't get rid of, but it was winter. I was a new mom, exclusively nursing, and just thought I might have postpartum depression, because it started to be that I couldn't even get out of bed. My husband began to take off work because I'd beg him in the mornings not to leave. I was just so sick. We didn't have a car at the time, and I physically couldn't make it across the bay to where my doctor's office was. My son was getting sick because I was sick. I went to my son's pediatrician a few times for my own care. Finally, they gave me the strongest antibiotics they could and told me to go to the ER if I didn't get better in twenty-four hours.

"When I went to the ER, the guy who triaged me thought I was a drug addict because of my heart rate and swollen eyes. I was with my mom, breast-feeding my son, and eating some nasty food my husband brought up from the cafeteria when the doctor walked in looking like he was gonna cry. He told me I had leukemia. I had zero white blood cells left. I just shouted, '*Mom! Mom!* What's going on?' I got checked into the hospital, started chemotherapy the next day, and didn't go home for about a month and a half.

"Before we went to the hospital, the denial was thick for everybody. I knew I was too sick to take care of my son, but I didn't want to tell anybody. He had been waking up all the time to eat because he wasn't getting any nutrition from my breast milk. My gums were so broken down, I wasn't even really eating anymore. I was taking multivitamins as a substitute for food. After my diagnosis, they took my son from my arms, and I had to stop breast-feeding immediately. They gave him formula, and for me that was like somebody stabbing me in the heart. He looked over at me as he was drinking the bottle, and I could almost hear him saying in his own way, 'It's okay, Mommy.' It was a struggle the first few days when my parents brought him to visit. When they left, I went into the bathroom and screamed, 'They took my baby!' The doctors said he could stay there with me, but I decided it would be harder for me if he was there.

"In the beginning I really saw my doctors as saviors. I didn't have a chance to get a second opinion; they said I would have died that weekend if I didn't start induction chemotherapy. Chemo seems quite archaic; they are poisoning your body to make it better. With a stem cell transplant, they bring you to the brink of death by killing all of your own bone marrow, and then they give you life again. Realizing the brutality and inhumanity of cancer treatment has been the most shocking thing for me.

"Because I am Chicana and African American, they told me finding a stem cell donor was going to be hell on earth. I have some qualms with how they figure out who is gonna get a donor and who is not. They find a racial match for you, based on what you look like when you walk through the door. It is a very old idea of race. In America, our ancestral lineages are so mixed up. I'm part Creole African American, part full-blooded Cheyenne, and my great-grandfather was a white French guy—so how do you know what I am? It is true there are very few African Americans in the donor bank, and that is why my chances of finding a match were so slim. I had a weird twist of fate. My brother and sister, who are fraternal twins, were perfect matches. It's rare when a sibling matches you, so to have two was like winning the lottery. My brother was the donor. He fucking saved my life.

"I grew up with sort of hippie parents who didn't believe in Western medicine. Having leukemia gave me a new appreciation for science. I signed up for a clinical trial at Stanford. They asked permission to take extra bone marrow for their studies. I said, 'Sure.' It turns out that marrow pulls are really excruciating, like having a metal butter churn in your back. The nurse hadn't even told me what it would feel like. So that was when I realized for the first time as a patient, I don't have to say yes to everything.

"I've had some cruel things done to me as a research subject, people being overly aggressive with my body because I'm young. They'll say things like

"**My trial** was the only way I could afford treatment. I could've quit the day I got a clean scan, but if I got off the trial and my cancer came back, I'd never be able to get back on. So I took treatment much longer than I needed to just in case: two days a week for twenty-six months. I am one of the only remaining survivors from the trial and my chart is the thickest one they have."

—*Krista Hale, 39*

your kidneys can handle it, and then they blast me with some drug that knocks me on my ass. I feel disabled now; I'm going into meno-pause at twenty-six, I have quadruple vision, my hands shake all of the time so I can't paint any more. I don't feel that science has failed me, but I feel that it has been cruel to me. It feels very cold. You are poked and prodded. Because you are a number in their research, they want you to do well, regardless of your quality of life. Doctors simply see death as their enemy. If you have a heart-beat, that is what counts.

"**My testicular cancer** doctors said, 'You're gonna get right back to playing football and having a normal sex life.' I was like, 'Oh really, because I didn't do either of those things before cancer.'"

—*Brian Lobel, 23*

"I have had some very compassionate doctors, too, but I've also had ones that act like they are gods. We should only be grateful to them, and how dare we ques-tion them? I remember seeing a sign at a nurses' station that said, 'Angels at work.' How can you question an angel? How can you question a god? How can you say, 'God, why are you giving me this drug? God, why does my body hurt? You brought me back from the brink of death, God, but I don't feel good.' They tell us we won't feel any side effects, and then when we do, it is like we have failed. I started to realize if doctors are God, then there is no hope for me because I'll be so afraid to tell them when there is something wrong.

"My doctors underestimate my intellectual capacity. I'd ask my first doctor a question, and he'd say, 'We'll cross that bridge when we come to it,' and I'm like, 'No, fuck you. This is my body, I'll cross it right now.' One day he told another one of my doctors that he didn't feel like I was fighting. I'm laying in bed in pain every day. Who are you? You haven't gone through this. How can you measure what fighting is for me?

"Managed care is all about less time in the hospital. They throw you out, saying your fragile cells are less potent than an infant's, you could die if you get a common cold, but we're gonna send you home anyways because we can't afford to keep you in the hospital until you heal. This shifts all the responsibility from the hospital to the family at home, who has to stomach the burden of what happens if they get you sick. What if they give you something that's not sterile enough and you get a bacterial infection?

"Paul, our baby, and I are living in one bedroom in my parents' house, which has been an experiment, to say the least. Before cancer even came along, we were in tons of debt and thought this would be the best thing to do. I think we really underestimated what it meant to move back with your parents. There are now seven people living in their house. My brother's bedroom joins ours with glass doors. He's an adult too, so it's like we're all right on top of each other, one bathroom in the whole house.

> "It is nearly impossible to have a decent sex life when you are living with your mom and dad."
>
> —Katie Smith, 37

"My son's not allowed to go to day care because it could give me germs. So we are both at home. I want to live in a neighborhood where we can get out of the house, where I can walk to a park. I live in the 'hood literally—Bayview–Hunter's Point. It's dirty and very neglected by the city. I live on a street where they've shot cops, there's crack and prostitutes, and I wouldn't want my son walking around. We want to move back really quickly to the East Bay, but we don't have the money. We've sort of been thinking of creative things we can do, like house-sitting for a professor on sabbatical."

As Amilca spoke, I thought back to the drive-by shooting at my apartment building, in which my thirty-two-year-old next-door neighbor died on our door stoop from three bullets through his skull. During my first year of cancer, I lived in a studio apartment with holes in the kitchen wall and dank hallways with stained red carpeting from the 1940s. The water cut out intermittently for ten-minute intervals, usually when I was naked on the floor of the tub in a contortionist's position, protecting my bandages, while my mom poured water from a cottage cheese container to rinse the suds from my hair. She slept on a futon on the floor during my surgery and treatment and expressed in her quiet, polite manner that my apartment was a shit hole. It was what I could afford and to me it was home. It was my retreat from doctors' offices and hospitals, a place to hibernate, write, take long baths while listening to Patsy Cline, and plan my attack strategies for fighting the red tape of health insurance. I was able to drown out the neighborhood gunshots until my cozy cancer nest became yet another building in my daily life smacked by death.

Like Amilca, I, too, wanted to move from my firearm-plagued neighborhood, but unlike Amilca, I had emergency savings to fall back on and was able to make the move. Even if I hadn't managed to move to another apartment in a safer neighborhood, I always had the fallback of my worst-case scenario—moving across the country at twenty-eight to live in the guestroom of my parents' new house in suburban Pittsburgh. Amilca was already living with her parents. She had already resorted to her fallback, and it wasn't the safe middle-class home that my parents lived in.

Amilca continued, "I haven't quite figured out how to carve out alone time. My husband's tried to push me to do it because he needs to be alone, too. He's gonna lose his mind, especially living in a house with so many people. But I haven't really done it yet. I feel guilty sometimes if I try to take

> **"My nerves** were so raw from treatment that I couldn't stand to be touched. The contradiction between 'Don't touch me' and 'I love you' is quite humorous to me and my girlfriend now, but for the first year of our relationship it was a painful, annoying, impossible situation that just didn't make any sense."
>
> —Rick Gribenas, 28

alone time. I'm really isolated in my neighborhood so I can't go anywhere unless I ask somebody to drive me, and then I feel really bad. It's been really hard to figure that out.

"I've always known Paul was a nurturer, but I have been so surprised at his bravery. I don't know if I could be as brave as he has been, having to look at my son and think I may have to raise him by myself. Paul has literally been by my side every step of the way. He's the kind of man that will clean up your vomit or help you if you diarrheaed on yourself. He's had his own depressions and breakdowns, too, because this is fucking hard. Take all the crap that any new parent goes through and add death onto that.

"My husband is like a knight. He loves to sleep, but I remember him staying up all night in the hospital. He had a flashlight that he'd turn on to write down the name of the drugs and what time the nurses gave them to me. He made me feel safe at the most unsafe time in my life. I think for him it was probably a lot harder than he ever let me see. It makes me sad 'cause I couldn't be there for him because he was being there for me.

"When you get married at nineteen, you go through so many life transformations together. Right after he proposed, he said, 'What would happen if in a few years I want to dye my hair green?' We decided we should let each other dye our hair whatever color we want. It was a really immature thing to talk about, but I think we were saying something bigger, which was, 'If I go through major changes, will you still be committed to me?' Cancer has been the biggest one by far. We've become such different people. Paul can really accept that I'm never going to be Amilca the way I was before. That Amilca has died.

"In the hospital I was afraid I wasn't gonna be able to go back and be a mom again. Yesterday I said to Paul, 'I just want to take care of you guys.' I yearn for that, to be able to take care of them the way that I used to, to prepare lunch for them or sit up at night when my son's screaming and acting like a complete fool. I want to be able to say, 'I'm here.'

"It still is so hard for me to think about how I acted towards our son when I was in the hospital 'cause I think I rejected him in a way. I started to push him away so if I die, he won't be so used to me. It was something I felt like I had to do, yet it was still so painful to see him go home. Sometimes he'd cry, and it was like somebody pulling my heart out and stepping on it. I always thought of the quote 'To have a kid is to allow your heart to live outside your body.' I felt like they were taking my heart away every time they took him out of that hospital room, and I felt like I so let him down.

"Finally, this nurse Barbara (and I will thank her for this wisdom 'til the day I die) said, 'The biggest mistake would be to push him away. That will make him regret his life forever. If there's one thing you do, write a letter to your son, and if you're dead when he's eighteen, they'll give him this letter, and it'll mean the world to him. Tell him what you're going through. And if you're not dead and he's acting like an asshole at sixteen, you can say, "Here, this is what I went through when you were a baby."' I always hear that nurse's words when I start to get scared. I hear her say, 'Don't push him away.'

"My child was my motivation. During the painful procedures, I sometimes think, Well, Paul could take care of himself if I wasn't here, and my family could deal, but my baby's the one reason why I've let them put that goddamn metal, churning, torture implement in my ass. I'm like, Well, if it would give him a few more months with his momma, it's worth it, so get it together, girl, feel this and just go through it. He waited to walk until the week I got out of the hospital, which I was so happy about. He's really loving to me. I think he knows, he's so gentle sometimes with me.

"When I left the hospital, I couldn't touch my son because I had a big central line in. I had a big catheter hanging out of me; everywhere I'd go, I'm luggin' around this fluid. I can only eat special foods that don't have bacteria. Anytime I was outside, I had to wear a humongous, rubber HEPA filter mask. It makes you look like a praying mantis 'cause it covers the bottom half of your face so all you can see are your eyes. It's hot and you can't take it off. When I wore it, mothers pulled their kids away from me in the grocery aisle, a guy in Trader Joe's asked me if I was planning a terrorist attack, and someone else asked if the mask was because my kid stank too much. Paul'd get so frustrated, he'd yell things like, 'She has cancer!' That didn't make me feel any better. But he'd be my mouth because it was useless to try to cuss somebody out with the mask on.

"It's hard when you become the thing nobody else wants to be. When you have cancer, people are like, 'Oh God, I'm so glad it's not me.' Not everyone says that out loud, but even when it is unspoken, you can still feel it. In the crisis moment you're still a hero, but when you have to have somebody help you wipe your butt, you're not so interesting anymore. When you are frail and vulnerable, people wanna sweep you under the rug or pretend like you're okay.

> "**A girl tried** to take my virginity because she didn't want me to die a virgin during chemo. Very sweet of her, but it didn't work. I had been at the sperm bank three times that week and wasn't feeling very sexy."
>
> —*Brian Lobel, 23*

"I go to see this guru, Amma. I firmly believe she is the Divine Mother. I don't impose my beliefs on anybody. I'm not here to proselytize. But I needed this kind of meditation and knowing there is something bigger than myself in order to live in that damn hospital room as long as I did. Amma visits the United States but lives in India, where she just opened a cancer clinic. It is the most state-of-the-art hospital in India. It was inaugurated by the president. I want to go there to volunteer. I don't know if it will end up happening. I feel like I am being called to go, but it is a little scary.

"Before I had my baby, I worked as an education coordinator at UC Berkeley, where I went to college. After having my baby, I had no real career plans. And now I see my new role in life as being a patient advocate. I feel like it is my gift to give, and I have been called to serve. I walk into a hospital, and opportunities abound. One day when I was at the hospital, I saw a woman who spoke very little English and was crying because the doctors wouldn't listen to her. I sat with her a long time. In many ways, we are in the same boat. Death is the great equalizer.

"There are people who have been on this cancer path before me, and they have made some grooves in the road where I can settle my feet down. I thank them for that and want to do the same for others. I don't want to save anybody. I know you can't do that. I just want to sit with people. I remember the immense loneliness and think that just sitting with someone can be very powerful. In this way, I think of my cancer as a gift because I'm very hard-headed, and I think cancer knocked me on my ass and is forcing me to get some important shit done in this lifetime that I wasn't going to do any other way.

"I'm not interested in charity. I want to selflessly serve. True service is getting rid of that illusion that there's any difference between you and me. It is the willingness to be humble, to let someone yell at you sometimes 'cause they are in pain or have them tell you they want you out of their room. You have to be careful not to take away people's humanity when you serve them. It is easy to see someone as weaker than you, and, physically, cancer patients may be very weak, but we know that they're not weak at all.

"The cancer world is the world I'm choosing to live in versus just walkin' around and being with 'healthy' people. The hospital is my world still. When you have leukemia, you live in the hospital. I started to see home as a vacation. It's not like I want the hospital to be my whole world, but that's my community now, the cancer community. It's where I feel the most comfortable, which is bizarre to me 'cause I never would've thought of a hospital as being comfortable. And it's not really the hospital, but I'm used to sick people. I like being around them. It makes me feel not so alone. It's going to be an interesting next few years of my life. Instead of being lost in treatment, I have to get lost in living."

Amilca and I walked outside and found Paul and their son asleep in their parked car. Because of germs, we did not hug but looked long and directly into each other's eyes. As she climbed into the passenger seat, Paul awoke and thanked me deeply for giving Amilca this quiet time to just talk. Toward the end of our time together, Amilca had told me that her chances of survival were 20 to 30 percent. I was glad I hadn't known those numbers at the beginning of our conversation. I feared that I would have asked her questions about mortality and her son with an uncomfortable sense of urgency or preciousness. As I stood in the middle of the street watching their car pull away, I shuddered to think that I could have done what I so often loathed in others: treated someone else's cancer with coy gestures and kid gloves.

> "**Ambiguity is more** real than a prescribed prognosis, which is complete crap. If there's an 80 percent chance of this, or a 20 percent chance of that, it's still a chance. Who knows which percentage I'll fall into?"
>
> —*Rick Gribenas, 28*

RESOURCES

Clinical Trials

Clinical trials are viewed as a gateway to receiving the most cutting-edge treatments available. Great news, unless you are a young adult. Although we are able to participate in many clinical trials for the eighteen to sixty-five age range, don't exhaust yourself trying to find trials exclusively for eighteen- to thirty-nine-year-olds; virtually none exist yet.

Although over 60 percent of all pediatric cancer patients are taking part in clinical trials, only 2 percent of twenty- and thirty-something patients are in clinical trials. Our lack of participation in clinical trials is partly responsible for our stagnant survival rates as compared to pediatric patients and older adults.

Get Clinical

To answer your questions about clinical trials, read "Clinical Trials: Questions and Answers," available from the National Cancer Institute, www.cancer.gov, 800-4-CANCER (800-422-6237). This fact sheet will help you understand what a clinical trial is, how one operates, and the pros and cons of participation.

The Extra Edge

Dr. Archie Bleyer, a champion of adolescent and young adult oncology, is leading the efforts to make clinical trials more available to young adults. Go online to read the table "Barriers to Participation in Clinical Trials" that Dr. Bleyer wrote for the book *Cancer Medicine* 6 (Hamilton, ON: BC Decker Inc., 2003). This list is an excellent tool for troubleshooting and overcoming your own potential barriers to clinical trial participation. Do a Web search for "Barriers to Participation in Clinical Trials" and "Bleyer."

Tracking Down Trials

Tell your doctor if you are interested in participating in a clinical trial, and be persistent. Oncologists are notorious for overlooking young adults as participants in clinical trials.

- Ulman Fund Clinical Trial Matching Service, www.ulmanfund.org, 888-393-FUND (3863). Clinical trials are listed under the "Services" section of the Web site.
- National Cancer Institute, www.cancer.gov, 800-4-CANCER (800-422-6237). Under "Clinical Trials," click on "Search for Clinical Trials."

- ClinicalTrials.gov is a comprehensive registry of federally and privately supported clinical trials conducted in the United States and around the world.

Family Matters

I placed in front of my living room window the most rigid, hard-backed chair in my apartment. For an hour I stared at the sky with the phone receiver molded to my sweaty palm. I finally called my parents and told them I had cancer. Many twenty- and thirtysomething cancer patients I have met describe breaking the news to their parents, their kids, or their siblings as the hardest part of their cancer experience.

Parents of Young Adults with Cancer

The Ulman Cancer Fund for Young Adults, www.ulmanfund.org, 888-393-FUND (3863). Receive parent-to-parent support via the Survivor and Loved Ones' Network. Read the downloadable booklet "No Way: It Can't Be: A Guidebook for Young Adults Facing Cancer," chapter 6: "A Parent's Perspective."

Cancer in Young Adults . . . through Parents' Eyes, www.cancerinyoungadults-throughparentseyes.org. This book and Web site just for parents provides advice and many stories from other parents. Add your own story to those collected on the site.

Ten Tips for Parents

From Diana Ulman, the chair of the board of the Ulman Cancer Fund for Young Adults and the mother of a three-time cancer survivor:

1. Find ways to help your child without overstepping or hovering.

2. Assist with time-consuming tasks that may be overwhelming to your child: record keeping, researching his or her disease or

body-mind medicine, or cooking healthy meals to store in your child's freezer.

3. Talk openly about the level of involvement your child wants you to have in his or her medical process.

4. Make sure that conversations with doctors are not directed only to you but to your child, too.

5. Try hard to let your child maintain as much independence as he or she has become accustomed to.

6. If your child moves back home, talk about what you each expect from the experience and how the rules might be different from when he or she last lived with you.

7. Be upfront with your child and ask questions about how he or she is feeling; don't try to read your child's mind.

8. Try to have some conversations that don't focus on cancer or on how your child is doing and feeling.

9. Stay strong for your child and don't let your emotions affect him or her; find a friend, a counselor, another parent, or another outlet where you can vent and cry.

10. Give yourself a break from thinking and talking about cancer.

Parenting with Cancer

CancerCare for Kids is designed for the cancer patient who has young children and for teens whose parents have cancer. It offers publications, online and telephone support groups, phone counseling, education workshops, and limited financial assistance for child care. Parents with younger children can download the booklet "Helping Children When a Parent Has Cancer." Parents with teenage children can download the fact sheet "Helping a Teenager When a Parent Has Cancer." To access these and other

CancerCare for Kids resources visit www.cancercare.org and select "I am a person with cancer." Then click on "Specialized programs" and choose "CancerCare for Kids." Or call 800-813-HOPE (4673).

Kids Konnected provides cancer support and education to parents with cancer and their children and teenagers. Visit www .kidskonnected.org or call 800-899-2866 to locate support groups, e-mail a therapist, find camps, and read what other kids and teens are saying about coping with a parent's cancer.

Love Sick: Teens Reflect on Growing Up with a Parent Who Has Cancer is a full-color, fifty-page anthology of poems, essays, stories, and artwork created for and by teenagers whose parents are living with cancer, which is produced by and sold through Kids Konnected. See contact information above.

When a Parent Has Cancer: A Guide to Caring for Your Children by Dr. Wendy Schlessel Harpham (New York: HarperCollins, 1997) comes with *Becky and the Worry Cup*, a children's book about a girl whose mother has cancer.

Myplanet.planetcancer.org. This social networking site for twenty- and thirtysomethings with cancer has an active online forum on parenting with cancer where you can dish with others who know what it is like to be a mom or a dad with cancer.

Sibling Resources

Witnessing my cancer was a frustrating and gut-wrenching experience for my thirtysomething brother. A void exists for resources that can help siblings of twenty- and thirtysomething cancer patients. If you are a sib in this age range, break ground in this new terrain by creating a Yahoo group, a blog, or a Web site to give and get support.

5

Malignant and Indignant

I ran through Potrero Hill with street maps falling from my bag, late to meet Geoff. My mind was stuck on a comment my father's best friend, Mike, made to me: "You'll never get a guy to talk to you about his cancer. Guys never talk about their feelings. I'm telling you it won't happen." I started arguing with Mike in my head as I zigzagged down the sidewalk. "I don't need anyone to talk about his feelings," I defended. "I'm not a therapist. It's just conversation, and plenty of men are happy to talk about their experience."

But what if Mike was right? Was I headed for a long session of trying to extract details from Geoff, where silence would be an aggravating itch and I'd stammer on like an idiot about my own cancer, hoping that he'd follow my lead? Would he sit there staring at me blankly, or I at him? This was starting to sound more like a date, and then it struck me, What if he's hot? What if he's hot, single, and thinks I'm hitting on him or that the whole reason I wanted to meet with him or even write this book is to meet a guy with cancer, who will understand what it's like to love someone who is ill and has a weakened immune system and can't go into smoky bars on dates? What if that *is* the whole reason I'm writing this book, to find a guy who will understand my feelings? But guys don't have feelings, according to Mike. So I was off the hook. I found myself ringing the buzzer to Geoff's guitar repair shop, which is a pretty hot profession, if you ask me.

Geoff answered the door, and as I extended a handshake, he greeted me with a hug that gently plucked me from my hyperactive mind and located me back in the convivial cradle of the Bay Area. Although Geoff was handsome, with a cyclist's frame—wiry, muscular, and thin—I was focused on what I had traveled there for: his story of long-term survival.

Geoff led me to the tiny back room of his guitar repair shop. We sat down, nestled between a small fridge and his collection of racing bikes that dangled from hooks on the ceiling. Geoff perched on an old kitchen chair, with his hands resting gently in his lap. He maintained a posture and pacing that were even-keeled, practical, and relaxed. We entered into conversation with more ease than I had with any of the women I'd met. Like a seasoned expert on living in the skin of death, he spoke thoughtfully and without a moment's hesitation. Geoff had been diagnosed with angiosarcoma at age twenty-two and been given six months to live. That was thirteen years ago.

"I shouldn't be alive. I have a greater chance of being struck by lightning than of sitting in this chair right now. I should be floating on cloud nine, absorbing the beauty of every moment, but I'm not. Sure, my experiences have changed me, but there's still the tedium of day-to-day existence. You read books about people getting cancer and nearly dying, and they're saying, 'I was enlightened, and

I suddenly saw the world with clarity.' I've spent thirteen years wondering what's wrong with me—why don't I see the world that way? And I've finally realized that there's nothing wrong with me. We've got human brains. They've been programmed for years. Having cancer isn't gonna suddenly make me the Buddha.

"**The only change** cancer has made in my life is I now splurge for a Coke with my meal instead of just drinking water."

—*Brian Lobel, 23*

"When I was twenty-two, I'd been living in Norman, Oklahoma. I had a really hard time: drug issues, a felony conviction, run-ins with the law. I'd just graduated from college and was in a pretty negative space, so I decided to get student loans and go to welding school. I started getting abdominal pains that felt like I had just been kicked in the crotch all day long. I saw a doctor who said, 'No, I don't feel anything. You just have an infection. Don't sweat it, you're twenty-two.' One doctor ran a blood test that had suspicious counts, which in hindsight could've definitely been scrutinized more carefully, but, you know, I was so young, everybody's operating under the assumption that I'm healthy. I went to a few different doctors, took antibiotics for a month or two, and the pain got worse and worse. I took a whole bottle of Advil just to make it through the day.

"**If I had** breast cancer instead of sarcoma, people could say, "Oh, my mom had that," "My friend's wife had that." I was surrounded by people but felt very alone because nobody had heard of my disease."

—*Chrissy Coughlin, 34*

"I got out of welding school, went up to Nebraska, and worked for a week. I woke up one morning and thought, Something is *so* wrong with my body. I called in to work and said, 'I'm done. Good-bye.' I threw my stuff in my car, drove right back to Oklahoma, and went to my urologist. This time he felt something, did a biopsy and CT scans, and found that I had angiosarcoma that had metastasized to my lungs. I went into his office and asked my parents to leave. I just asked him, 'What's the deal? The real deal, not the bullshitmake-the-parents-feel-good deal.' He put his head in his hands and said, 'You know, it's just really bad. A guy your age. It's just a tragedy.' The doctors told me that I might have six months.

"My parents dealt with things pretty well. My dad was able to get me on his medical insurance policy with only two days left on the window of eligibility. My mom got me to MD Anderson Cancer Center in Houston, and within a couple of days I was on chemotherapy. MD Anderson is the cancer factory; they just roll you through. When I walked in there, I saw people with catheters hanging out of their faces and just knew this was serious shit.

"I also immediately realized that at Anderson, I could get whatever kind of pharmaceuticals I wanted. I had done drugs since I was ten or eleven years old. My childhood and teenage years were a lot of turmoil, no discipline, no guidance from my parents. I had already been to drug treatment when I was seventeen. At Anderson, I could pretty much just say, 'This is what I want,' and I got it. It was like ordering fries at a drive-thru. I think they just figured, 'Let's give him anything he wants, I mean, he's gonna die anyway.' I was taking tons of Xanax, morphine, and Marinol—synthetic marijuana.

"I was in and out of the hospital for a year, and during that time, a lot of relationships fell away. Very few people stuck by me. My family couldn't even talk about it, and most of my friends couldn't deal with it, either. I was so absorbed in sickness, I didn't realize at the time how hard my cancer was for others. I just thought, Well, why can't they come and hang out with me? When my friends and family did come, they'd act like nothing was wrong. It was very fake. It almost felt like a viewing. They'd stand up against the back wall and just look at me.

"When my younger brother came to the hospital, he really hung out with me. He was very different. We just talked about normal guy stuff. He just accepted me. What I most wanted was a sense of normalcy and for somebody to say, 'How's it going today?' Not 'How's your cancer?' or 'How's treatment?' I wanted my friends and family to say, 'What's on TV? What are you doing?' 'Cause even though there's all this new shit going on with your cancer, there's a person in you who still wants to have fun and wants to live and not have everything be so heavy all of the time.

"Dying of cancer in real life is not like in the movies, where a group of people circle your bed saying, 'He was such a great guy.' I thought, If everyone knows I'm dying, they're all going to come in and say, 'I really enjoyed having you as a friend,' or 'I wish we could have done some things differently in our relationship, but I love you anyway,' and that just didn't happen. People don't want to accept change. They think if they pretend everything is the same, it will just be that way. I pretended, too. I had this legacy of just being a fuck-up, and I didn't feel like I really had the right to hold anyone account- able. I don't feel that way now, but at the time I did. I guess we all might have been doing the best we could do.

"After six months, I went back to Oklahoma and stuck to the chemo regime that MD Anderson laid out. I was in remission, but we knew that I could come out of remission even while still on chemo, it was that aggressive. I was sick all of the time, but I was still trying to lead this facade of a normal life. I lost thirty-five pounds and often slept sixteen hours a day, but there were also times that I still felt like being active. I was going out with my friends, going to bars. I'm drinking, just partying like crazy, and looking like death. I was really out of con- trol. My doctors were just placating me, giving me chemotherapy and whatever other drug I wanted. I tried to have this normal life, yet I'm dying of cancer.

"I had a chemo port installed in my chest and was supposed to lie in bed for two weeks with the port under my skin. Instead, I went out mountain biking two days later. If I hadn't been on so many drugs, this never would have happened 'cause the pain would have been too great. I was totally jarring my upper body. Then I crashed my car. I almost killed myself, and instead of getting help, I just got out of the car, and I changed the spare tire myself. I jacked the car up and everything, with this port sewn into my chest.

"When I went to the hospital for my next round of chemo, the doctor opened up my shirt and was like, 'Oh, my God! It looks like a Doberman has been chewing on your port. We can't use this.' He grilled me, 'What happened to this site?' I just responded, 'I don't know.' I guess this is the difference between being an old man and a young guy with cancer. It's like, 'I'm gonna go mountain biking, and that's just how it's gonna be.' I was mentally thumbing my nose at being sick. That time was definitely not all about me trying to live, 'cause I think I was actively trying to kill myself, too."

As Geoff spoke, I listened hard, as if my heart was straining to pop out of my ears. I physically ached to hear more of his story. Although the details were painful, I craved the truth of his harsh and destructive cancer experience. I had grown tired of images of cancer patients smiling with gratitude. I cringed when I heard stories of strength and hope, not because they aren't important or real, but because I experienced a flip side that is never spoken about. I experienced the lowly jones for something to cut away at my pain and fear. These were not beautiful moments. They have not become the subject of talk shows and do not make a good photo shoot for a cancer walk-a-thon poster. I had become resentful of the pedantic stages of grief that describe anger as a hoop to jump through on the road toward cancer enlightenment. Geoff's desperation was acrid, and no thick coat of finesse or grace could paint it otherwise. I was glued to his every word as he told his story.

"Soon after the incident with my port, I actually coughed the tumors out of my lungs. It was really weird and pretty unheard of. My oncologist was shocked. I guess he expected that I would have kept them in a baggie or something. I'm like, 'Sorry, they're in the Circle K parking lot.' He was furious because he wanted to study them, but the thought never even crossed my mind. I was like, 'Dude, I thought I was coughing up a lung. I mean, if it helps you at all, I can tell you that they kind of looked like chicken livers.' I was just so sick and so out of it. My world was all about chemotherapy and drug abuse. My family was like, 'Not only is he dying, but he's also a disaster zone.' How do you approach someone like that? It's impossible.

"Back in Oklahoma City, I was in the hospital one out of every three weeks. The chemotherapy was so caustic, they had to give me a twenty-four-hour IV that coated the inside of my bladder so that I wouldn't rot from the inside out. When I was in-patient, my narcotics were all administered by nurses so I couldn't take the really high doses I had been giving myself. I started waking up out of this fog of drug abuse. One night in the hospital, it was two or three in the morning, this older guy and I were pushing our pumps up and down the halls, and we started talking to each other. He had worked at the air force base for a long time with toxic metals. He had a bunch of different cancers and was gonna die. While I was listening to him, I just realized right at that moment—I'm not going to die right now. I just thought, I have got to change my life. I can't live this way anymore. Whatever time I have left, even if it's just a couple of months, I am not wasting it.

"The next day, still dressed in my gown and pushing a pump, I took the elevator from the fourth-floor chemo ward up to the seventh-floor drug treatment center and checked myself in. I had been there in high school when my parents made me go. This time was really different. I was ready to be there. My goals were so simple: all I wanted was to live the rest of my life without hurting anyone else.

"I did in-patient drug treatment for a month, then I lived in a three-quarter-way house for a few months, all while I was still taking chemo. After I sobered up, I decided, I'm not taking chemotherapy anymore. I don't want to live the rest of my life being a slave to medicine. Even if I come out of remission, I don't want to live my last few months in the hospital. All the chemo, the illness, everything had just become too rough, and I thought, Fuck it, I'm not doing it anymore. I don't care if I die. It wasn't about quitting; it was about taking my life back, even if it was an abbreviated life. I feel like I woke up to the fact that I do have some choices. Deciding to take chemo at all or even to go to the doctor in the first place, these are hard and scary choices, but they are choices. I called my oncologist and told him I'm not doing chemo anymore. We talked, and he convinced me to take three more rounds of chemo, and I don't know if that was right or wrong for a doctor to do, but I'm still here so I'm not complaining.

"A month after my last round of chemo, I got a clean bill. It was weird because it's like, So what do I do now? I don't have any purpose. The whole year has been so intense, emotionally, mentally, physically, and then all of a sudden they pat you on the back, say, 'Good luck,' you're out the door, and then it's over. I felt like I had post-traumatic stress disorder or something. Everything just seemed so meaningless. I'd wake up and my days seemed totally intentionless, drifting by. When you have cancer and you wake up every morning, man, you know what's happening: chemo, scans, IVs, the whole protocol. Everything else just falls away. There's no confusion. Life was perfectly clear on chemo."

Geoff's words, midway through our conversation, became those of a teacher, and my attention that of a student. Unlike other young patients I had talked with, he had lived a prolonged cancer recovery that was free of recurrence. I hadn't noticed until speaking with him that I craved instruction on how to handle life after treatment. It is hard to be surrounded by illness and then suddenly be catapulted back into a world of work and hanging out with friends who still think they're immortal. Some days I wondered whether my quest to speak with other young cancer patients was slightly pathological, whether I had a problem letting go of being in the cancer world, and whether maybe this book was just an extended visa that allowed me to stick around a while longer. I asked Geoff how he shifted back into his work and social life.

"I tried to achieve some sense of normalcy in my life, but it was hard. I found some welding work at a bike shop. A lot of people recovering from cancer talk about trying to live life like there's no tomorrow, but you have to work, you have to go grocery shopping, you can't just walk around 24/7 thinking, I have to make the best of it because I could die in the next five minutes. It's not realistic. We all know we're going to die someday, it's just that people with cancer have gotten a little taste of it. That doesn't make us different from anyone else; we all walk around with the same potential for living or dying or being happy or sad. I think there is a lot of expectation placed on people with cancer to be hopeful, but I was really lost. I had no idea what to do for myself, let alone how to give hope to other people.

"I was always seeing my life through this lens of: I'm going to die. I really wish someone had told me, 'Don't hang on to that bullshit. Move forward. Don't sit around thinking that you're going to get cancer again 'cause at that point you're already dead.' I've been posing this heavy

"**I've wanted** a tattoo of a phoenix if my scans work out but I never celebrate any of my good news. Every time I get good news I feel like the hammer has just been held up a little longer."

—*Nora Lynch, 24*

"**There was outside** pressure to be a Superwoman and work through all of my treatments because so-and-so did, or so-and-so ran a marathon during cancer. For me it was a no-brainer: I'll go back to work when I'm ready and not until then. I have great benefits and I'd be stupid not to take advantage of them."

—*Jill Woods, 38*

philosophical question to myself: If the doctors came to me and said, 'Your cancer is back and you're going to die tomorrow,' would I look back on these past ten years and say they were worthwhile or would I say I've fucking blown it? I've been struggling with this question for over a decade, and the struggle itself has kept me from really living.

"Once you've had cancer, people like to think of you like a superhero, like Lance Armstrong, but I'm no superhero. I don't go for that image. Cancer recovery has become so romanticized, as if this one event suddenly made me a whole different person. I don't think that's the case.

"I've finally realized that I don't need a big label like 'survivor.' Everyone thinks that survivors are fighters. I don't think I really fought for my life. I laid there and got doped out of my mind for six months and got well, while other people were sitting around reading Bernie Siegel, doing their imagery work, and died. Nobody can say they should have fought harder. What does fighting mean? Maybe some people who are super-fighters are completely afraid but can't admit it. Are we just focusing on the fight? Is 'survivor' a term only reserved for the people who make it, for the people who don't die? And are the people who make it then just survivors? Survival is bullshit. I don't want to aspire to be a survivor. I think it's my big 'survivor' story that I've been telling myself for ten years that has kept me at arm's length from my own life.

"I'm no superhero, and I don't want to be one. I don't think my body got rid of my cancer for any heroic or noble reason. I won't ever really know why my body beat these crazy odds, but I have my own theory. I think I got better because my body was so used to processing drugs. I was a drug addict. My body knew what to do with chemicals, and it knew what to do with chemo. Just me sitting here is so unlikely. There's no answer.

"I don't know what really cured my cancer or what really caused it. The common thread through angiosarcoma patients is industrial workplaces. I had been working as a welder and hadn't worn a respirator. Maybe I was inhaling a bunch of heavy metals, who knows? Maybe I was genetically predisposed, and the metals kicked it off. I haven't thought that much about where it came from and why. I don't think most people do. Instead, we are just focusing on a cure, not the cause. Maybe the cure needs to suffer a bit so the cause can be addressed. We should refocus our thinking. I mean seventy thousand young people a year get diagnosed with cancer. Where's the outcry? Where's the outrage? It's not happening. It just seems like there are a lot of words out there about cancer, but they're just words. I saw a girl standing in front of the Indianapolis airport with her yellow Live Strong bracelet smoking a cigarette. I thought, What the fuck are you doing? What does that mean to you? Is it just some little trinket? Money got put to a cause, but as far as raising people's awareness, I don't know how deep it goes.

"I began going to a young adult cancer support group about a year and a half ago because after thirteen years, I finally felt like I had something to give back to others. My mom was like, 'You've made it so far, you've done so great, you've really suffered and struggled, and I don't see why you need to go back and do all that.' I went to a group meeting last night, and it's true that there are some really sad stories, but these stories are still there whether I turn my eyes away or not. At this point in my life, I don't want to turn my back on someone else's suffering.

"When I first started going to the group, I thought that if I reopen this chapter of my life, I'm gonna get cancer again. And I do

> "**I stayed** at Hope Lodge during my transplant and I played the piano every night. The other patients loved listening and were glad I wasn't someone from the outside playing the flute or giving weaving lessons, making them feel all sick and pitiful."
>
> —Brian Lobel, 23

> "**I chose** to resign from a new job and collect unemployment. I took writing classes and did all the things I never had time for. How many people in their seventies and eighties look back on life and say, 'I wish I had worked more?'"
>
> —*Debbie Ng, 27*

assume that I am gonna get it again some-day, just as a side effect from all of the treatment. It's very scary. I'd be completely lying if I said it wasn't, but over the past years I've had time to get okay with the fact that I'm mortal. That's just the way it goes. Nothing I can do about that. All I can do is live and try to be good to other people 'cause I'm not gonna cheat death. And that's the thing I want other people with cancer to know—that even if you think you're gonna die in six months, or you got this shitty prognosis, or your life's a fucking wreck, it's never too late to turn around and say, 'I'm gonna figure out how to live the way I want to live.' It's just never too late. Yeah, I know I sound like a Tony Robbins seminar. And I know there can be some really dark days, but I'm confident that if my cancer comes back, I can deal with it. I managed to deal with the intensity of cancer twelve years ago when I was walking around messed up on drugs with a pump hanging out of my side, and I know if I had to, I could do it again. I'm not particularly fearful of death, but it's so easy to say that right now. I'm sure I'd feel a little different if I got a lump in my arm tomorrow."

My conversation with Geoff lasted only three hours, the shortest one I'd had so far. I don't think it was because he is a guy or that he had less to say. He was busy leading a life that wasn't focused 100 percent on cancer but instead on running a business and racing bikes. Geoff's returning to a support group and listening to our gory cancer stories in the middle of his long-term survival was beyond admirable. People had started to ask me how I could bear to listen to other patients' pain after what I had gone through with my own can-cer. It was not always easy. Sitting with someone else's real suffering and pain made it concrete that recovery is anything but graceful and revealed that cancer patients are not heroes. We are simply people trying to manage and outsmart pain and fear. We are normal people who are trying to live.

I ended my San Francisco trip with a visit to my surgeon. He recommended biopsies of my suspicious neck nodes and operating if they were positive. To an objective ear, this would have sounded like a routine response, but I'd just spent four years anxiously awaiting a clean bill of health. Even the hint of more surgery or treatment felt like receiving my original diagnosis all over again. I added to my map of San Francisco new landmarks where I cried on my cell phone to my mom and friends: a falafel shop, the Best Buy parking lot, and a hillcrest in Pacific Heights while I watched slow-moving cargo ships haul heavy loads under the Golden Gate Bridge.

Back at my Chicago hospital, I asked the intervention radiologist to measure my nodes before performing the biopsy. When he said the largest was seven millimeters, I hopped off his operating table and explained that through my own research, I learned that biopsies of neck nodes less than one centimeter yielded inconclusive results. I used the grueling and inconclusive biopsies he had previously performed on my small nodes as supporting evidence. Why should the insurance company and I pay for a biopsy that would suck up blood and no tumor cells? Why should my family and I wring our hands awaiting pathology results that would return inconclusive?

I hurried upstairs to my doctor's office and in an unscheduled appointment proposed a plan born not of medical expertise but of my own simple logic: I had one of the slowest-growing forms of cancer, nodes that were too small to biopsy and could either be malignant or merely benign nodes reacting to a cold, PMS, or a skin blemish on my neck. If a repeat ultrasound in six months revealed that they had shrunk, the chances were that they were not cancer, and if they had grown, they would be sizable enough for a biopsy. My doctor, who was nearly at retirement age, had never treated a patient in this manner. A bit dumbfounded, he saw no holes in my argument and conceded to my plan. I drove home feeling like nobody's fool and wondering when the medical world had abandoned common sense.

RESOURCES

Employment Issues

In case you aren't challenged enough by figuring out what to make of your $80,000 college degree or how to work your way up the career ladder while starting a family, fasten your seatbelts for this sobering statistic: Americans who are actively receiving cancer treatment are laid off five times as often as other workers. Sucks, huh? So, how do you not become this statistic?

Educate yourself about cancer in the workplace. Strategize before disclosing your illness. Research before writing your résumé. Role-play before your next interview. Doing so will greatly increase your chances of getting and keeping the job you want and creating a more friendly work environment. Remember, you are not alone. There are more than 10 million cancer survivors in the United States, many of whom are returning to work, and 80 percent of those who worked before cancer return to the workplace after treatment.

Employment Rights and Wrongs

Use these resources to educate yourself on the Americans with Disabilities Act (ADA), the Family Medical Leave Act (FMLA), short- and long-term disability, how to disclose your illness to an employer, minimizing your chances of workplace discrimination, reentering the workforce, job hunting, self-employment, rebuilding and maintaining your finances, and more.

"Working It Out: Your Employment Rights as a Cancer Survivor," written by Barbara Hoffman, JD, and published by the National Coalition of Cancer Survivorship. Download it at www.canceradvocacy.org, or call 877-NCCS-YES. (877-622-7937) for a free hard copy. Scour the Web site for other excellent employment information.

"Off Treatment: Financial Guidance for Cancer Survivors and Their Families." Download it from www.cancer.org or call 800-ACS-2345 (800-227-2345) for a free hard copy.

Cancerandcareers.org is a treasure trove of information targeted to women, but the content is applicable to men, too. Be sure to check out its "Ask a Career Coach."

Short- and Long-Term Disability

Enlist the help of a social worker or legal advocate to see if you qualify for various forms of short- or long-term disability compensation that will allow you to receive income while you are not working. See Lean on a Legal Advocate on page 27.

Résumés and Disclosure

Whether to disclose your illness to an employer and how to hide gaps on your résumé depends on your personality, your communication style, your field of work, the size of the company, and the perceived atmosphere of the workplace in question. Seek the help of a social worker with extensive experience in career counseling for cancer patients or people with disabilities. Work together to create an individualized approach that reflects your career goals and work history. CancerCare is well-known for its counseling on employment issues; visit www.cancercare.org, or call 800-813-HOPE (4673).

Finding and Keeping a Job

- Make short-term and long-term job goals: short-term career goals at a second-choice job can help you pay off medical debts before you venture into achieving your more satisfying, long-term career goals.

▪ Believe in your capabilities. Feelings of inadequacy can be a barrier to success in an interview or in the workplace. Seek professional counseling to talk about boosting your confidence.

▪ Know what you are going to say in an interview or to a current employer and/or to coworkers before they are given the chance to ask. Practice your answer outloud, make your explanation brief, and end on a positive note by enforcing your skills and what you bring to the job.

▪ Never lie on a résumé, in an interview, or on an insurance form because it can lead to automatic termination.

▪ Wait until after a job offer has been made to ask about health insurance. Refer to it as an employee benefits package, rather than as the company's health insurance plan.

▪ If you have a disability plan, make sure that returning to work will not require you to forfeit your benefits. With Social Security Disability, investigate the Social Security Work Trial program before you return to work.

▪ If you are self-employed and carry individual health coverage, thoroughly research all health insurance options before making any changes to your current coverage.

Peer Support

Does the phrase "support group" conjure up visions of Kleenex, metal folding chairs in a circle, and a therapist relentlessly thanking you for sharing your feelings? Ditch those notions of old-school support, and end your isolation by diving into a plethora of new support options exclusively for young adults with cancer, most of which were created by young adults with cancer.

Get Connected

MyPlanet, myplanet.planetcancer.org. Planet Cancer is a social network where users provide irreverent, candid, and meaningful peer support. Create a blog, post in the forum, share photos and videos, start a group, and connect with others in your area.

I'm Too Young for This, www.i2y.org. Go online to find your local chapter, and participate in happy hours, regional young adult cancer conferences, and other events in your area for young adults with cancer.

Stupid Cancer Show, www.i2y.org. Listen to this weekly, interactive, online talk-radio show hosted by i2y's Matthew Zachary.

Waiting Room Magazine, www.waitingroommagazine.com. This online publication is the only magazine for young adults dealing with cancer. Its haute design is delicious eye candy.

Get a Group

CancerCare's online and phone-based young adult support groups are moderated by the savvy social worker Julie Larson. In-person young adult groups are also available in the New York area. Visit www.cancercare.org, or call 800-813-HOPE (4673).

Locate young adult support groups and networking events near you:

- Check out the listings on www.ulmanfund.org by going to "Home," then clicking on "Services," followed by "Support Groups."
- Consult the calendar of national events on the home page of myplanet.planetcancer.org.
- Search online for a support group in your area that may not be listed on either of these sites.
- Call hospitals in your area to see whether they have groups for young adults. Often, you do not need to be a patient at a hospital to attend its support groups.

Get a Friend

With many young adults in their databases, the following organizations will try to match you with another young adult who has your type of cancer, to share experiences and give support. Imerman Angels also excels at matching young adult patients with similar life circumstances, such as matching college students or patients with young children.

Imerman Angels, www.imermanangels.org, 312-274-5529

The Leukemia and Lymphoma Society, www.lls.org, 800-955-4572, First Connect Program

The Ulman Cancer Fund for Young Adults, www.ulmanfund.org, 888-393-FUND (3863), Survivors & Loved Ones' Network

Get out of Town

Planet Cancer, www.planetcancer.org, 512-452-9010. An organization for young adults with cancer that leads retreats including re-orientation weekends, kayaking for couples, and spa retreats for young adults.

First Descents, www.firstdescents.org, 970-845-8400. This organization offers kayaking and climbing adventures exclusively for young adults with cancer.

Camp Mak-A-Dream, www.campdream.org, 406-549-5987. Check out the retreats for eighteen- to twenty-five-year-olds.

Real Time Cancer, www.youngadultcancer.ca, 709-579-7325. This Canadian young adult cancer organization leads the annual weekend-long "Re-Treat Yourself" retreat, as well as an annual young adult survivor conference.

I'm Too Young for This, www.i2y.org. This Web site has extensive listings of excursions and retreats nationwide.

Get Real

If you have received peer support and want to give it back, help by ending the isolation that many terminally ill young adults face. Twenty-two percent of twenty- to thirty-nine-year-olds with cancer will not survive. Get real with this fact by offering yourself up to conversations about death and dying with peers who will likely not make it. Spend time visiting, calling, and sending e-mails or cards, even if they are too ill to respond. Read about end-of-life issues on page 131 and from other sources to increase your knowledge, chip away at your own fears, and learn how to show your presence, love, and support to this often invisible part of the young adult cancer community.

6

Something in the Air

In the months following my California trip, I uncovered a gigantic cancer taboo: admitting the fact that having cancer does not necessarily make someone a nice or interesting person. On a regular basis, I was held hostage for hours on the phone by boring or whack-job cancer patients who wanted to meet me: a fuming young West Coast real estate agent with cancer blathered about twelve-step meetings, the housing market, and the relentless challenge of hiring a good personal assistant; a droning twenty-three-year-old testicular cancer patient itemized the aerodynamic features of his new bicycle and helmet—purchases inspired by Lance; a thirtysomething woman with breast cancer ranted hysterically from a coffee shop in Harvard Square, admitted she was off her meds, and disclosed to me her child-hood incest; and a twentysomething woman dragged on a cigarette while relating the downright incongruent details of her cancer story (I suspected that her ailment was actually Munchausen's syndrome). No matter how tedious, melodramatic, or maniacal these people are, how do you cut off patients who are seeking to confide in you about their cancer? My pathetic solution was to trigger call waiting by calling my landline from my cell phone. I'd say that I needed to take the call and that I'd contact them if I would be traveling to their area.

I could afford to lose a few hours in my week to the whack jobs because my phone calls and e-mails from cunning, down-to-earth cancer patients more than made up for it. I was happily receiving unemployment, spending most of my time researching young adult cancer statistics, and deciding from a growing batch of promising new contacts whom to meet next. While in California, I had lengthy cancer conversations with a filmmaker in San Francisco and a gutsy singer-songwriter from Los Angeles. Back in Chicago, I spent an afternoon talking with an installation artist. Subverting the emerging pattern of meeting with creative and artsy patients, I decided to scout out the complete opposite for my next cancer conversation: a straightlaced, full-time business professional who was a Bible-quoting, Christian suburbanite.

Meanwhile, I attempted to reverse the same trend in my dating life by placing a moratorium on artists. As I sat across from lawyers, engineers, and real estate agents in tapas bars and French restaurants, Wafa'a's words echoed through my head: "When I date guys who are really together, they make me feel undone." I didn't know which sounded worse on a date, having cancer or being a choreographer on unemployment. Writing this book was both my greatest alibi and my largest detriment. My dates were fascinated by the project but always asked what led me to write about young adults with cancer. "Helping my best friend through her cancer diagnosis and treatment," I lied. Some men called my bluff immediately, and others silently waited until I came clean a few dates down the line. Their rejections ranged from

"I have kids and don't want to bring something like cancer into their lives," to "My dad had cancer, and I don't think I can go through that again," to an optimistic "This must be a really stressful time for you. Maybe we should just be friends and sleep together."

On my second date with a guy named Shannon, we were sitting on his couch when I grabbed the remote and turned off *The Daily Show*. My head was about to explode. I couldn't stand it any longer. With most men, a container of raw cookie dough and a weekend of watching *Sex and the City* cured me of their rejections, but in only a date and a half, I was so taken with Shannon that I knew a sympathy rejection from him would push me over the edge into abject heartache. "I have something really important to tell you," I prefaced. I told him I was living with cancer, stressed my high cure rates, and omitted the atypical behavior of my case. "Okay, we will deal with it together," he responded. He was loving and empathetic about my cancer and confessed that he felt slightly relieved because he had feared that my breaking news would be an announcement that I was dating someone else. I was stunned. Shannon had released the pressure valve on four years of cancer dating angst. The moment reminded me of waiting for test results that actually come back as good news but you want to cry anyway from all the stress of waiting. I held back my tears of relief in effort to not look like an overly emotional cancer freak.

Shannon and I became glued to each other's side. He fervently learned about contemporary choreography and asked for daily debriefings on the cancer statistics I was researching at the library and online. I was equally curious about his work as a nonprofit environmental lawyer defending the clean air and water acts. Many of the young cancer patients I talked to questioned why researchers did not focus more on the environmental causes of our disease, and I asked for Shannon's help in finding the answer. He introduced me to his coworker Richard Acker, a thirty-six-year-old environmental lawyer with stage IV colon cancer. Richard also happened to be a straightlaced, suburban, Evangelical Christian.

Richard lived with his wife, Karen, and their ten-month-old daughter in a split-level ranch so pristinely kept that I could see vacuum tracks on the carpet. Warm and inviting, the Ackers made me feel like an important guest in their home. Karen left with her daughter to run errands, giving Richard and me quiet time to talk in the living room. Unlike every other twenty- and thirtysomething I knew (myself included), Richard did not constipate his sentences with "like," "um," and "you know." His speech was eloquent, as if he were reading from an edited journal.

"This may sound weird, but I've had a lot of joy in my illness because I've seen the wonderful things it has caused people to do. Friends from church, from Karen's old workplace, and neighbors baby-sit while we go to doctor appointments. We are also blessed that our parents live in the area. People from church mow our grass and helped plant almost five hundred plants in our garden. When Karen and I receive help, it is clearly benefiting us, but it also gives some benefit to those who are helping us. They feel good. It makes them happy. It helps them to express their love for us in a concrete way.

"I believe that there are times when it is appropriate to receive help, just as there are times when it is appropriate to give help. If you ever refuse to receive, you are unnecessarily putting a barrier between yourself and the love of others. It's normal for humans to live in communities where there is love and relationship, and receiving is just as important a part of being in that community as giving is. It is happier for us to be supported and uplifted by others, rather than being alone wrestling with something very hard on our own and saying, 'I'm not going to share this cancer struggle.'

"I've had friends say, 'Richard, it's not fair that you would get cancer. You are young; you have a young child; you are doing good things. Someone else should get cancer, someone whose life is not as productive.' My feeling is, fairness doesn't enter into the question of who gets cancer. The Bible says the rain falls on the just and unjust alike. There is no one person who is more or less deserving of cancer than any other.

"I don't think that God sent the cancer. I think that bad things don't come from God. They come from the fact that we live in a fallen world where there is sin and disease and death, and God uses these bad things and turns them into good things. So perhaps the reason 'Why me?' is that God sees a good opportunity to be glorified through me. If, for example, God gives me a miraculous healing, I plan to talk about it. I plan to say, 'God did something great in my life.' If I can bring people to faith and can open up their eyes to the magnificent character of a loving God through that, then that was totally worth it. My cancer will be used for good, despite the fact that the cancer itself is a bad thing, and if given the choice I would certainly choose to not have it."

Richard's words brought ease to my chronic existential struggle of parsing out the good and the evil in cancer. Being a black-and-white thinker since birth, I had refused to see any good in my cancer for fear that someone would dare to interpret this wretched disease as a gift. But I had experienced positive moments: watching the outpouring of love during treatment from my parents, brother, friends, and cousins who lived so far away; sharing deep, meaningful conversations with this growing group of cancer patients across the country; and learning that I had the smarts to comprehend complex medical information and challenge my doctors. Sitting next to Richard, I recognized that no matter how hard I tried to separate the two, the piss and the stink

> "**I don't think** there is any reason I got cancer. I don't think it is because I deserve it, or am going to learn from it. I think it is bad luck, bad genes, or a toxic environment."
>
> —*Jill Woods, 38*

of cancer do exist side by side with cancer's goodness and gifts. I thought, Maybe this is why cancer hurts so much, because the good and the bad are so heightened, close to the surface, and constantly ricocheting off each other. Maybe cancer wouldn't be so horrific if the evil of our illness experiences was sealed off in a distant vacuum, far from the reminders of what makes life pleasurable and worth living. As I listened to Richard, I did not need to believe in God, miracles, sin, or heaven to find deep meaning in his words.

"Part of my character is when I am faced with something, I want to examine it from every angle and turn it around in my hands and comprehend everything about it. With cancer, you can't; there are too many unknowns. My prognosis is not certain. The extent of the disease is hard to determine, even the best scans only give you an approximation. Things come and go without explanation. I try to understand what I can to make informed decisions about my treatment, of course, but I recognize my limits and know this is something I will never be able to grapple with entirely, and I'm not going to knock my head against a wall trying. Instead, I will take the elements that are beyond my control and turn them over to God—which is both scary and comforting. It's scary for me to let go of something, but it is also comforting to say, 'God, you could control this, so I leave it in your hands.'

"I have moments of fear where I can envision Karen crying and me not being there to give her a shoulder. I can imagine Karen going to her parents or to her friends from church to seek consolation because I'm not there. I have times when I can imagine my daughter being six or seven years old and saying, 'Where is Daddy?' To me, those are terrifying thoughts. I let them pass through me. I try neither to reject them nor to obsess over them. They come and they go. When I have those thoughts, I feel an overwhelming desire to live. And when I have those thoughts, I pray.

"Praying is like having a conversation where you just open yourself up to God and speak to God like I am talking to you. I say,

'God, you know what I am facing, I don't have to tell you, but it helps me to talk to you. Please work a miracle, because the doctors don't expect me to get cured.' They say the median survival is twenty months. I say, 'Father, what we can do here on earth is pretty limited, so I need a miracle of healing. You created everything, so this is pretty trivial in comparison.'

"I fear being dead, but I don't fear dying. I don't want pain, but in the end, big deal. I can deal with pain, and they can give me drugs. It is not being here that would bother me. What bothers me is Karen coming home to an empty house. The idea of my child going off to college and doing great things, and I am not there by her side to congratulate her. That is what really bothers me. That is what I fear, what Karen fears, and my parents, too. They say that one of the most stressful things that can happen to a parent is to lose a child. I fear for the hurt for those who would be left behind. For me, it won't be so bad. I get to go to heaven. One of the biggest reasons I want to live is to save my family from pain and loneliness. If I die, I don't know what good would come out of that pain and suffering and sorrow, but I also know that from our perspective as mortals trapped in time, we don't have the ability to see the good that can come out of something like that."

Richard excused himself to help Karen. She had returned home with their baby in her arms, coughing and throwing up from the flu. The sounds of water running in the bathroom and fresh baby clothes being pulled from dresser drawers reminded me how incredibly simple and singular my life with cancer was. How Richard had the energy to work eight-hour days—even on his laptop when he was receiving chemo at the hospital—and still have time to manage his

"**People at work** say how strong I was and they couldn't handle cancer if it was them. I probably thought I couldn't handle it either, but when you are faced with it, what choice do you have?"

—*Jill Woods, 38*

medical care, rest and eat well, and spend quality time with his family was incomprehensible. When he returned, I asked about his work as an environmental lawyer.

"Speaking as an ignorant layman, cancer is a broad rubric for an incredible variety of diseases. Cancer is complex by its physical nature, where the cells divide so rapidly that you can't get a handle on them. Not many other diseases are like that; most others retain the same characteristics throughout the disease. They don't go through ten generations within your body so one medication starts working and then stops. It is somewhat discouraging that we haven't made more advances against cancer, other than early detection and treatment, but it is also not surprising since its rapid reproduction makes it so hard to nail down.

"In an industrialized society like ours, we are putting huge amounts of chemicals into the environment and into our bodies. We do not know the long-term effects, especially synergistically. More and more studies are showing one to two hundred synthetic chemicals in the average person's bloodstream. Did you know the average person has fire retardant in their bloodstream because of all the cushions we sit on and the clothes we wear? The FDA, the EPA, no one has ever studied the effects of these many chemicals together. Each chemical is thought to individually pose a minimum risk, but what if you have one hundred and fifty things that are each individually minimal risks, but perhaps three or four of them combined might cause a greater risk than we have ever learned about? On the other hand, some believe that in industrialized societies, as health care improves, the older you get, the more people will get cancer just because that is what happens to human bodies as they get old. They become more susceptible. I am in no position to make a judgment on that. But it is a note of caution to society that probably everyone who reads this book has dozens, potentially hundreds, of chemicals in their bloodstream, and the cumulative effects of those are unknown. Could they be causing cancer? Maybe, I don't know. There is that chance.

"Part of the reason they don't do the research on cancer and chemicals is because the chemical companies don't really want them to. And the federal government is not particularly enthused either about researching things that could cause economic impact if they were withdrawn or restricted. But also it is partly just the difficulty. You do the math. If you have one to two hundred chemicals, in order to research the potential effects of the combination of each of those, if you take a pair of every three or four of those chemicals, there would be hundreds of thousands of potential experiments. It would be totally cost prohibitive. And to do it on a large-enough scale where you could get statistically significant results, how could you do that? It would be extremely difficult, so I don't totally blame industry or the government for not doing it. But the truth is, the consequence of the expense and the reticence of not doing this testing is that the whole American population is in a sense guinea pigs for the effects of dozens of synthetic chemicals being put into the human body. That is just reality.

"One of the principal motivations for choosing my career as an environmental lawyer is I have always keenly felt the beauty of the world and a desire to protect God's creation. I feel that beauty even more acutely now because I realize that my perception of it may not last as long as I expected. When I see a beautiful night sky, I realize I don't know when I'm going to see that again. When I see the cardinal flowers blooming in the spring, I think I'll probably be here next spring and the spring after that, but I'm not sure. So I feel a greater urgency to appreciate these things immediately, while we have them."

> **"People want to know** what caused my cancer because they want to figure out how to not get what I got."
>
> —*Greg Dawson, 36*

I asked Richard to talk about his belief in God and Christ. Being an evangelical, he was more than happy to oblige. For an hour and

"**I've spent** much of my life reading, studying, theorizing, and cancer made me want to go out and feel, touch, taste new things. I'm more adventurous with food, more into getting hugs, I go to the petting zoo more often, but it's not like I'm doing ecstasy or having sex in bathrooms."

—*Nora Lynch, 24*

a half, he shared with me his faith in the Gospels, views on the relationship between God and man, the history of the Bible, and the origins of life itself. He and I could not have been more opposed in our theological beliefs—or lack thereof in my case. Prior to cancer, this conversation would have launched from me a thousand sharp rebuttals. Sitting in Richard's living room, however, I noticed something different in me. I wanted to listen more deeply and considerately to his beliefs even though they were so contrary to my own. I saw clearly that since cancer I had become significantly less judgmental, and the process of writing this book in some ways served as my platform for testing out this newfound ability.

RESOURCES

Cancer and the Environment

Growing up as teenagers in Pittsburgh, my friends and I hung out in the secluded wonderlands of abandoned steel mills and mountainous slag heaps. Although the toxic playgrounds of my youth were extreme, many young adult patients I've met reflected on childhood memories and asked, "Did using my microwave, eating BBQ, or my summer job on a farm cause my cancer?" And, "What in my current environment might still be contributing to my cancer?"

Think Green

The resources below provide sound information that will educate you rather than simply inciting enviroparanoia.

"Cancer and the Environment: What You Need to Know and What You Can Do." Download this free booklet or call for a hard copy. National Cancer Institute, www.cancer.gov, 800-4-CANCER (800-422-6237).

The University of Pittsburgh Center for Environmental Oncology (www.environmentaloncology.org) for consumer-friendly brochures and fact sheets on household toxins and other tips to help you lead a healthy lifestyle. The Web site also offers more advanced articles from peer-reviewed journals.

"State of the Evidence: What Is the Connection between the Environment and Breast Cancer?" Read this report issued by the Breast Cancer Fund and Breast Cancer Action. A PDF is available for download on the Web sites www.bcaction.org and www.breastcancerfund.org.

Building Support Systems

During my second treatment, I received assistance from an organization whose volunteers help with household tasks. Instead of vacuuming or walking my dog, Nancy spent her volunteer hours online scheduling fifteen of my friends and neighbors to run my life. Without my even having to ask, they arrived at my home like magic with clean stacks of laundry and food for my fridge.

A Little Help from Your Friends

Asking for help is time consuming and emotionally exhausting. Remove yourself from the equation by finding a reliable friend or family member with stellar admin skills (someone other than your primary caregiver) who can coordinate your needs using the following tools.

Lotsa Helping Hands, www.lotsahelpinghands.com. This free, easy-to-use, private online group calendar allows friends, neighbors, family, and colleagues to sign up to help you with daily life tasks. It includes pages for messages, photos, links to maps, and space for specific notes about your medications, food desires, and more.

Share the Care: How to Organize a Group to Care for Someone Who Is Seriously Ill (New York: Simon & Schuster, 2004). With practical tips, task lists, and troubleshooting techniques, this book is the best resource for learning how to organize and maintain a well-functioning care group.

Hire a Pro

Educate yourself about different levels of home help, how to find home-care services, the appropriate questions to ask when hiring an agency or individual providers, and various ways of paying for or having home care covered. Visit the American Society of Clinical Oncology Web site, www.cancer.net. Enter the Patients, Families, and Friends portal. Select "Coping" from the left-hand menu. Then choose "Caregiving," and finally "Home Health Care."

For most young adults, home health care is not covered nor is it an affordable option. If you still desire some home help with basic household chores, consider asking friends to skip out on buying you flowers, teddy bears, and pink ribbon trinkets, and suggest that they instead chip in twenty bucks to your home helper fund. If you cannot afford a home help agency that prescreens workers, ask through the grapevine for referrals to a trustworthy nanny or personal assistant who could use some extra cash. If you are organized with your to-do list and find an energetic helper, even using someone two hours per week can make a big dent in your errands or light housework.

Best Support-System Secret

Simplify scheduling and buy more home-alone time by making copies of your house key or using an outdoor lock box, so that friends and helpers can stop by to clean or drop off food while you are out.

7

Mortality Bites

I turned my living room into a mini cancer library. Hundreds of white index cards plastered the walls, all scribbled with resources, statistics, quotes, and contact information from young adult cancer patients. I planted my desk in the center of the room, and up around it grew towering stacks of cancer magazines and journals, research studies, and booklets from the National Cancer Institute and grassroots healthcare organizations. I was addicted to checking e-mail, eager to hear from new cancer patients. One Friday evening, while heading out the door to a dinner party, I couldn't resist the last ding of the day and opened

"**Most days** I think I don't want to die yet. And other days I think if I went right now my life will have been a really good memory."
—*Amilca Mouton-Fuentes, 26*

an e-mail from Amilca. It had been sent by her husband, Paul, to Amilca's entire address book, to let us know that she had passed away.

Bundled in my winter coat, I sat in shock at my desk. I cried as threads of drool dripped onto my keyboard. I felt as if the index cards hanging on my walls were quaking with laughter, scoffing at my naiveté, at how utterly shallow I was traipsing around the country and chatting with young cancer patients about death and dying as if it were a subject matter and not an actuality that would sooner, rather than later, happen to some of us. I had so ignorantly assumed that the only people in this book who would die were going to be the patients I had yet to meet with in hospitals or hospices.

Mourning someone I had met only once for four hours felt like an act of trespassing, as if I were sneaking into the backyard of those who were grieving the loss of Amilca as a wife, a mother, a daughter, a sister, a friend. Though it sounded trite and clichéd, I kept thinking that the world was a worse-off place without her in it. I didn't mean worse off in the metaphoric sense but in the tangible sense. There were things in this world that Amilca was going to do to make it a better place. She had an agenda, and it was everyone's loss that she was no longer around to fulfill it.

With Amilca's death, I felt deeply why saving the lives of young adults really, really matters. Although no one deserves to or should die of cancer, and it seemed vastly uncouth to say that any age group has more of a right to live than another does, I thought it anyway. Society had invested two decades' worth of education and resources in Amilca. She was a skilled and caring mother, a literate and quick thinker, a compassionate and moralistic person. I wanted the world to reap the benefits of that investment for decades to come.

Seth Eisen was familiar with the process of witnessing a young brilliant person be snuffed out by cancer: he had watched his thirty-three-year-old brother die of melanoma. Seven years after his brother died, when Seth himself turned thirty-three, he, too, was diagnosed with cancer. While I was living in San Francisco, Seth introduced himself to me backstage after one of my performances. We sat in the empty theater, gabbing into the small hours of the morning about cancer, friendships, family, and relationships. We immediately became each other's cancer confidants. We attended a young adult support group together from time to time, but our best conversations usually happened at each other's kitchen table.

I had wanted to record a conversation with Seth since the inception of this project, and I took him up on an offer to join him in Philadelphia when he flew back east to visit his family. Our meandering discussion occurred over two days in cafés, on the train, and in my hotel room.

Seth began, "My brother's death was an awakening for me. For me, cancer was the C word at that point. I had to dispel a lot of fear around the C word. I finally realized that cancer can be a vehicle for transformation, even if it means death.

"I really looked up to my brother as a role model. He was smart and successful. He paved the road for me coming out of the closet and being an artist. After graduating college, I moved to San Francisco to be with him. From the time I was teenager, he was so supportive of me, and when he was diagnosed, it was my time to be there for him. I resigned from my job and asked my family to support me so I could be his primary caregiver. I didn't know what the fuck I was getting into. I was navigating doctors, being his friend, and being with him through extreme bouts of anger, frustration, and all the things you go through in the process of dying and accepting your demise. It was a really difficult time. There was so much suffering. He really didn't want to live as long as he did. After he died, I found all these books on euthanasia under his bed. He bought

> "I told my mother
> I don't want a big costly funeral when I die. People think it is morbid to talk about but you should think about these things ahead of time."
>
> —*Krista Hale, 39*

them, thinking, If it gets really bad, I want to kill myself, I don't want to suffer. I wish he had communicated that with us because in the end he couldn't talk, he couldn't tell us what he wanted.

"**I tried** to act okay even when I wasn't to keep my parents from breaking down and worrying about losing another kid to cancer. I joked a lot because if I was serious I knew I'd break down."

—*Krista Hale, 39*

"The last thing my parents needed after losing a son to cancer in such a horrible way was to see another son of theirs going through treatment. When I was diagnosed, I just begged them not to come. I was like, 'My partner, Keith, is here, I have a strong community. Come visit when I'm done with chemo and radiation.' They said, 'Tell us when, and we'll be on a plane the next day.' I was so glad they weren't insulted. I just couldn't bear having to see them see my brother in me. I needed to go through this on my own with every bit of positive energy. Plus, let's face it, my parents and I have very different lifestyles; they are very religious and I'm gay.

"There were other ways my parents could help, besides being here physically. I was happy that they engaged their community in praying for me and sending me cards. They helped me out financially. When I was losing my mind and couldn't function, I could call my mom and have her walk me through how to boil an egg.

"I grew up in a culture of service. My family was very generous, even though they had small means, and everything they taught us was always about giving to other people. My biggest lesson with cancer was learning how to receive. Here I am, this thirtysomething guy, I thought I should be able to support myself, take care of myself. Who cares what is wrong with you? Just get your shit together and find a way to take care of yourself. That is how I always thought you were supposed to do it. I suddenly needed to change from a person who just tried to take care of himself to a person who invited my community to help me.

"Keith was organized and practical. He sat down with me and asked, 'How much money do you need? How many months might this take? What kinds of help do you need to make this successful?' I needed rides to chemo, people to make meals for me and do my laundry. I needed money. I had just left a job, and while I qualified for disability, my COBRA payments were huge. I had a roommate, but my rent was still expensive. I wanted to see a therapist, an acupuncturist. I had co-pays for tests, doctors' visits, and medication. I made a chart of what I needed, and I broke all of these costs down. I wrote nice and clear e-mails, saying, 'If you want to donate money to a good cause this year, you can donate it to me; I'm a good person to keep on this planet, and I want to survive cancer.' If I didn't ask, I would not have gotten the money. My friends also threw a big benefit for me at this swank little downtown gallery club and raised five thousand dollars.

"**I think** in ten or twenty years they will think chemo and radiation are barbaric, like the iron lung. But for now I need to trust myself to these proven treatments rather than drinking grass juice and following medical advice from an infomercial."

—*Jill Woods, 38*

"The thing I most want to tell people in their twenties and thirties is find your community and ask for help. Even if you feel isolated, try to organize. Most people want to help you but don't know how. A perfect example of this is everyone and their freaking grandmother calling me up and saying, 'My Uncle Joe had cancer and oh my gawd, this spirit gum tea from Mozambique is just the best thing, and it is going to cure your cancer, too.' I got five thousand of those kinds of phone calls and was ready to just puke. It's not actually helpful. So you need to clearly state what your needs are and recruit people to take care of them. I had a gathering of friends before my treatment.

I wrote down all the weeks and different tasks on a sign-up sheet. It made things really smooth. People really came through. I could see how much they wanted to help."

Seth's story reminded me of how strongly people reacted to the well-organized network of friends that ran my life during treatment. Many friends were thrilled to be part of something that felt like a community. They thanked me for allowing them to help and enjoyed meeting my other friends, who constantly came and went from my house. But others cringed, commenting, "Oh, I could never ask people to do all of these things for me. I'm way too private and independent." They made me feel as if I was a lazy prima donna sponging off my friends. I wanted to ask, "How would you go about taking care of your daily needs if you were single, living alone, had cancer, and your family lived twenty five hundred miles away?" Instead, I passively absorbed their disdain. At times, I allowed it to erode my confidence and cause me to question whether cancer necessarily robs you of privacy and independence. Weren't there other ways of doing it? Aren't there people who prefer getting their own glasses of water on their deathbed? Am I weak for not being one of them? The shame-laden debate raging in my head ceased as Seth spoke about where he had learned his lessons on forming a community around illness.

"I think being queer affords me a different perspective on cancer. Through the AIDS epidemic, not only have gay men come together as a community and shown our humanity, but we have given a gift to society by showing that we as a

> "**Being in a lesbian** relationship, some people acknowledged my girlfriend as my caregiver and others did not. We are domestic partners and I'm listed as a spouse on her insurance card, but our pharmacy still wouldn't let her pick up prescriptions for me. Instances like that add complexity to cancer."
>
> —Debbie Ng, 27

group of people know how to take care of our own. Do you? It might not be obvious, but during the worst part of the AIDS epidemic, my community learned to take control of their disease, make empowered choices about their illness and treatment, and said, 'Hello, U.S. government, we really need the drugs and we need them now.'

"It's kind of a bummer if you are a gay man with cancer in San Francisco. People automatically think it is HIV-related. My brother was also gay, and I remember when a hospice nurse came to the house and was like, 'Is this where the AIDS patient lives?' It's like, 'Read your goddamn chart, bitch.' It happened numerous times with my brother. I started wondering why it infuriated me so much. I realized it's because I am so AIDS-phobic. It's like, 'Oh, if you have AIDS, you must have done something terribly wrong. You've ruined your reputation as a human.' Screw that, too. Just because I've had cancer doesn't mean I can't get AIDS, too. I'm frightened of having another disease and know that as a sexually active gay man, I could still contract AIDS. I know people all of the time who do, even though they thought they were practicing safe sex. When I was going through cancer, I had an HIV-positive friend who would say, 'It's an all-out war, girl: cancer vs. AIDS. Now we're gonna see who wins! Who will live longer, me or you?'

"When my brother died, I joined a grievance support group. This group of people and I had nothing at all in common. I was the only gay person. We were different professions, races, socioeconomics, but we learned there is an immense amount of healing that can take place between

"**I'm not out** to my parents, so they think of my girlfriend as just my roommate. My cancer is allowing my family to see a side of her that they wouldn't have otherwise. They see how important she is in my life and what a wonderful person she is to me, even if they don't know she is my girlfriend."

—Debbie Ng, 27

people who are otherwise totally unrelated. Their pain was directly connected to my loss. That experience convinced me of the magic of support groups, so after I was diagnosed, I sought out a young adult cancer support group in San Francisco.

"Nobody there was gay, and people certainly had specific experiences of their own that I wasn't going through, but, regardless, every time I went, I still felt supported. Some nights the support group was not that inspiring, but it was still good to go because there is nothing like being around a group of people who are your same age and going through what you are going through. You are not going to get that kind of understanding from your doctors.

"I called my doctor's office every day. They told me to call them whenever, they didn't mind. I was on prednisone, which is like really intense speed, probably like being on crystal. You are on fire. I was so sick and feeble, couldn't even walk, but I also couldn't sleep, not even with sleeping pills. I was mentally out of control. I became manipulative. I was either crying all the time or laughing hysterically. The doctors and nurses realized I was like a speed freak, and they were nice about it, but they kind of said, 'You signed up for this because you want to live. You're a grown man. Just deal.' Their job requires that they not be reactionary or hook into your mental trips.

> "**I was terrified** of give myself injections. The nurses were like, 'Don't be a pussy' (not in those exact words). The first time I shook so hard I couldn't position the needle, but after a while I felt really tough, I'd turn the lights down low pretending I was in a heroin dive. I feel proud like I could do anything now."
>
> —*Nora Lynch, 24*

You go in, they spew out the info about what is going to happen to you, and that's it. My general practitioner told me that oncologists are good at what they do, but they are a cold breed, and they are not going to hug you or hold your hand. My oncologist is really brilliant and even had cancer herself, but her attitude was like, 'Let your family or boyfriend deal with your whining.'

"I remember waking up one night to a bright full moon, and everything around me just felt so real. I said to Keith, 'Honey, I think I am going to die tonight.' I was at my edge, and the Seth I knew couldn't go any further because there was just so much pain. It was like a spiritual death because I didn't know the person who was functioning after that night since every ounce of energy I had left towards surviving was gone. I didn't have anything left to give. I was at the end. I was past the end. I had so much sickness, so much neuropathy, I felt like I was literally disappearing. I was doing everything in my might to keep myself alive. I didn't lack the will, but I just didn't have any energy.

"At the end of treatment, I got super-sick with really high fevers from a rare infection and was in the hospital. They didn't know what was wrong with me. And I felt like I had already died. I remember seeing our friend Loren Olds on the floor of my hospital room writing checks for paying my bills, and I thought, It is over. This has got to be it. I cannot stay here anymore. I'm ready to die. I had a constant flow of tears. That is where I connected into what God and spirituality are. It is the brokenheartedness of feeling complete desperation. My heart was cracked open, and there was this incredible tenderness inside. Everybody has this tenderness, we just don't know how to get there. This fragile state is the closest to being at one with God or the universe. That vulnerable and raw reference point is the greatest teacher. That is where the Dalai Lama, Mother Teresa, and the really compassionate people of the world are coming from. They have a constant access to this deep understanding of what it is to be human and what it is to experience pain.

"To me, this is the most real place, but it's raw and uncomfortable, so why would you want to go there? We do everything we can in our power to run from that painful, ugly place. It is not necessarily

"**I have** a really big fear of dying so I've never let it enter my mind. I didn't get any tactics on death as a kid. My family's not religious. I've never even been to a funeral.

I was raised that if there is something bad you just push it away, and I think believing everything will be fine really does help in my healing."

—*Melissa Sorenson, 25*

what we would think of as positive. But it is real. We rush around our lives wanting happiness, but it evades us because we are not willing to touch what is real. We think, Oh, it is money or success or things being a certain way that will bring us happiness or satisfaction. But I think it actually comes from that brokenheartedness, which is our true humanity. It is the place where we are our weakest and our strongest. From that place, you can relate to anyone.

"I think, culturally, we want to turn our backs to what is really truly human, which is that you are fucking going to die, and it could be really ugly and painful, and your experience is really temporary here, and it is not pretty all the time. But I have way higher highs in my life now because I've seen this sadness and brokenheartedness. I think if you find the ability to hold these paradoxes, you actually have more of a capacity to live fully and to cope with the fact that life is full of paradoxes like this.

"After I went through this experience, my doors were thrown wide open and my guard was down. You think about your cancer experience hundreds of times a day. You feel you are different. You see you are different. I was pale, I had no hair. For someone in their thirties, you know, we are still workin' it. We don't want our looks to go down the tubes. And then there are people who say, 'God, you look great,' even though you feel like shit, and you want to smack them. It's really hard to let people know what you've just been through. People have an image of what it is supposed to be like when you are done; you're supposed to come out a saint. But I was so severely depressed. Here I am, a person with a master's degree, I've made progress in my career, then I'm gone for a year and a half, and I'm back to lifting boxes. Fuck that.

"I moved out of the loft I lived in when I was sick. I needed to divorce myself from that environment. When I drive by there now, I don't think of the five years that I lived there. I think of the one year that I had cancer there. You ask yourself, How much are you going to hold on to that identity as a cancer person and how much are you going to have a new identity emerge?

"Now, four years after treatment, I think about cancer once or twice a day. It's like a wound that has mostly healed, but it is like a gold medal, too. I'm now an authority on going through a cancer experience. At the time, I wasn't able to laugh at any of it. Now I kind of look back and think, What a clown I was, what a big deal I made out of everything. Carrying on and on.

> "**I continue to** discover things about my illness experience four years later, not because I'm not over it but because I'm still trying to wrap my head around it."
>
> —Brian Lobel, 23

"I do feel that people don't know me until you know I've had cancer. My whole identity is wrapped up in having gone through this really difficult period. There was always the question of, Am I separate from the disease or am I the same thing as my disease? Interesting question but unanswered."

Seth and I had been friends for four years, yet there was much I learned about him in those two days that I had not known before. Included in our marathon of nonstop talk was a trip to Seth's child-hood home for dinner with his mom and dad. They lived in a modest duplex, brimming with murals and paintings that Seth had made in high school and college. I was the first friend Seth had brought home in almost ten years, and his parents treated me like a queen, feeding me overflowing portions of home-cooked food. His mother and I bonded in the kitchen while washing dishes. She told me stories of all of her children, whose photos hung on the fridge. She spoke longingly about Seth's brother, how much she missed him, and how it broke her heart when Seth was diagnosed. "I've never been the same," she said.

After dessert, his mother announced that we were all going out dancing. "Your father never dances. It's been decades," she said in her thick Jersey accent as we piled into the car. "You kids will love it." In a dimly lit ballroom dance studio on the second floor of a strip mall, the room divided into men and women learning the cha-cha. His mother pulled me aside.

"Kairol," she pleaded, "don't you think Seth would be so happy with a nice, intelligent Jewish girl like yourself? Look at him. He's so smart and adorable. Couldn't he be so happy?"

I took her hands and said, "He is happy and, trust me, if there is anyone who knows what happiness looks like, it is Seth."

RESOURCES

"Out" Patient

Are you in the closet? Have you recently come out? If so, are your family and friends more distant? Do you or your partner have experience navigating the medical system as an "out" patient? Because of these and other variables, young lesbian, gay, bisexual, and transgender (LGBT) cancer patients may face challenges that straight or older LGBT patients do not.

Extra Advocacy

Most young LGBT cancer patients do not have the luxury of time, access to a major metropolitan city, deep roots in the gay community, or the stellar health insurance required to search extensively for an LGBT-friendly oncologist. Perhaps you will be lucky and find that your oncologist is compassionate and attuned to the needs of LGBT patients. If not, recruit friends, nurses, social workers, and members from your hospital's patient representative staff to serve as your extra advocacy team.

Ask your team to be your watchdogs at your doctor appointments, to help you clearly state your medical needs, and to advocate for you during hospital stays. Watch for common biases that doctors may display toward LGBT patients including assuming that fertility, scarring, or the loss of a breast or a testicle is less important to an LGBT patient, and neglecting conversations about sexual function.

Research Your Rights

Same-sex partners may be denied the visitation or power of attorney rights afforded to heterosexual couples. Understand your rights in advance; do not wait for an incendiary situation to occur before you investigate them. If you are protected under government law or hospital policy, print a copy of the law or policy to carry in your wallet or purse at all times in case you need to defend your rights in the hospital or emergency room. Remember that remaining as calm and polite as possible during a dispute will increase your chances of getting what you want.

Visit the Human Rights Campaign Web site at www.hrc.org to determine whether your state protects visitation and power of attorney rights for same-sex couples. Select "The Issues" from the drop-down menu across the top and click on "Health." Select "Laws," then choose your state. If you are not protected under state law, call your local government and ask if county or city laws exist to protect same-sex visitation and power of attorney rights. Seeking the advice of a legal advocate may help clarify these complex legal issues. See Lean on a Legal Advocate on page 27.

If state, county, or city law does not protect you, speak with a patient representative or hospital ombudsman and request a copy of your hospital's Patient Bill of Rights to see whether these rights extend to same-sex couples. Then befriend the hospital administrator who assisted you and use their name in conversation with nurses and doctors who may act in violation of your patient rights.

Unfortunately, you may find yourself with no protection at all. In these instances, try to identify an LGBT-friendly staff member, such as a social worker. Introduce yourself and ask if he or she can act as your advocate.

Seek Support

LGBT patients may have social support challenges that heterosexual patients do not deal with. Body image issues may be intensified if your partner's intact body becomes a reminder of how your own body has been altered. You may feel added isolation within the cancer community if you are the only LGBT member in a young adult support group or the only young patient in an LGBT support group. You may have to field discrimination or biased thinking, such as straight female cancer patients who speak negatively about looking like lesbians because they are bald from chemotherapy, or people who suggest that if you are gay with lymphoma you must have AIDS.

- Connect with others who understand what you are going through. Participate in these online support networks for LGBT young adults with cancer:

  The Gay Men's group on myplanet.planetcancer.org.

  The Lesbian and Bisexual group on myplanet.planetcancer.org.

  The Young Survival Coalition's lesbian, bisexual, and transgender forum for young women with breast cancer on the bulletin board at www.youngsurvival.org

- Seek one-on-one support directed toward your needs. Ask a peer matching organization to match you with another LGBT patient (See Get a Friend on page 102). If you are searching for a therapist, interview potential candidates to see if they are LGBT friendly.

- Read cancer lit that reflects your stories and experiences, such as *My One-Night Stand with Cancer*, a breast cancer memoir by the lesbian author Tania Katan (New York: Alyson Books, 2005).

- Check out "Unique Issues of Young Lesbian and Bisexual Cancer Survivors," a transcription from the Young Survival Coalition's teleconference program, available at www.young-survival.org. Click on "YSC community" on the left side of the page, and select "Diversity." A link to the teleconference transcript is listed under "Programs."

Best Advice for Coming Out to Your Doc

Create a situation in which you feel empowered rather than vulnerable. The Human Rights Campaign suggests talking to your doctor at the beginning of your appointment, prior to the actual examination, while you are still fully clothed, and bring a friend or your partner along to be supportive to you.

End-of-Life Issues

Since Lance's balls and bike became public, we no longer speak about cancer in hushed tones. Yet although cancer may no longer be the C word, death is still definitely the D word. End-of-life issues and fear of dying are particularly taboo in the young adult community. While diving into these issues may seem scary, it can also be extremely empowering and ironically life affirming.

Throw Back the Curtain

When I talked with Julie Larson, the young adult program coordinator at CancerCare, she spoke about facing end-of-life issues with young adults:

"The diagnosis of cancer brings up end-of-life concerns and worries for anyone, regardless of what stage you are in or what your prognosis is. When young adults are truly dealing with the end of their life, there is a fear of even talking about it. Sometimes people can engage in what I call magical thinking, that if I talk about dying, then it means it is going to happen. This thinking keeps you from having really important conversations that value your life.

"It takes courage to sit down with someone that you trust and throw back the curtain and look at what you are scared of, what you are really worried about. This is when the tears really come. I tell people our tears are messages that tell us very important things about what matters most to us.

"Some people do have concerns about pain and discomfort, but most often the tears are about missing their life, about missing certain people or certain experiences. If it is about missing a girlfriend, boyfriend, fiancé, spouse, your children, we find ways to communicate these feelings so those messages will not be lost."

Supportive Care

Does the idea of hospice totally freak you out? If so, you are not alone. To enroll in hospice, a patient must agree to end curative care; this can be a serious deterrent for many young adults who do not wish to surrender their hope for extending life. A more palatable approach for us can be palliative care, also known as supportive care.

A palliative care team most often comprises a physician, a nurse, and a social worker. These practitioners excel at administering pain-relief drugs with minimal side effects. The assistance of a palliative care team can be of great relief and comfort to both patients and their caregivers.

- Learn how palliative care or hospice can be of help to you, how to locate a palliative care team, and the differences in insurance coverage for palliative care versus hospice care at www .getpalliativecare.org.

- For a side-by-side comparison chart of palliative care and hospice, visit www.caringinfo.org. Click on "Living with an Illness," and scroll down to and select "Palliative Care Questions and Answers."

- The Ulman Cancer Fund for Young Adults offers a booklet titled "No Way: A Guidebook for Young Adults Facing Cancer" that includes a section on "Facing End of Life." You can download it from www.ulmanfund.org.

- Read Coping with Pain on page 147.

Taking Care of Business

Prepare for the financial and legal issues that may accompany the end of life, such as financial management, funeral or memorial service planning, and creating a will and a living will. Use these resources to help you get started.

Visit www.caringinfo.org. Click on "Planning Ahead" for information and checklists.

Read *Be Prepared: The Complete Financial, Legal, and Practical Guide to Living with Cancer, HIV, and Other Life-Challenging Conditions* by David S. Landay (New York: St. Martin's Press, 1998).

Not Just for Tots

If peds are granted last-wish trips to the Magic Kingdom with Michael Jordan, shouldn't we be able to go to Tahiti with George Clooney or Scarlett Johansson? The following organizations grant wishes to terminally ill adults.

Dream Foundation, www.dreamfoundation.com, 805-564-2131

Fairy Godmother Foundation, www.fairygodmother.org, 312-573-0028

Making Memories Breast Cancer Foundation, www.making memories.org, 503-829-4486

Find Things to Do That Will Live on after You

You and your friends and family can find it extremely meaningful to engage in a project that will continue your legacy.

- Plant a perennial garden.

- Write a letter or make a video.

- Make a scrapbook, time capsule, or blog documenting your life.

- Create a fund in your name directed toward a cause that reflects your values and interests.

- Enjoy meaningful time with special people that will live on in their memories.

8

The Myth of Eternal Optimism

I used to love the luxurious sequestration of an airplane; jetting past puffy clouds was where I daydreamed the deepest. But I noticed on my flight to Birmingham, in tiny increments, claustrophobia began to close in on me. I broke into a cold sweat and counted the seconds between touchdown and the door finally cracking open. I sprang through the Jetway with relief. I was in Alabama.

A Southern hospitality superstar, Tracy Wiginton insisted on picking me up at the airport. She greeted me with a huge hug and a welcome basket overflowing with pink-ribboned paraphernalia and food and drinks for my hotel room. Tracy and I had felt an immediate connection on the phone when she called me one month earlier, after seeing my flyer at a young adult breast cancer group. She described to me how cancer had changed her from a happy thirty-seven-year-old, full-time working mom and wife into a woman wrought with anxiety and depression.

I expected to head straight to Tracy's home on the semi-rural outskirts of Birmingham, but instead she chauffeured me on a cancer show-and-tell tour of the town. We drove around the University of Alabama Birmingham Comprehensive Cancer Center; visited the Camp-Smile-A-Mile offices, where she volunteered for kids with cancer; and met with Dr. Kvale, a therapist whom Tracy saw for care and worked with side by side on UAB's Distress-Management Team. We chatted in the park for an hour, as they educated me on this newly emerging field within oncology that addresses the psychological, social, and spiritual needs of cancer patients.

Four hours later, we finally landed on her oversized living room couch with Chick-fil-A takeout. I was itching to record our conversation and relieved that her husband and son had not yet come home, as Tracy intimated that they were not too excited about her meeting me.

Tracy began, "When I was diagnosed, I was in shock and depressed. The hardest thing I've ever done in my entire life was telling my son. I only have the one kid—he is my world. I try to protect him, take care of him, love him, raise him up in a good environment. When I had to tell him, I felt like a piece of innocence was taken away from me and from him. Here my thirteen-year-old son is having to worry about losing his mother.

"I told him in the car on the way home from school: 'When I had surgery the other day, they found something. And I've got breast cancer. Do you know what cancer is?' He said they studied it in school. I said, 'I've got cancer, but it's going to be okay. We're going to do everything that the doctors tell me to do. I'm going to be sick, and I'm going to have to take some medicine that will make me lose my hair.' I told him if I needed to shave my head, that the three of us could do it together. I wanted to throw stuff like that in to kind of ease it for him. I let him know I wanted him to be a part of what was going on. I don't want to hide anything from him, but at the same time he is only thirteen, how much of this can he grasp? 'It'll be okay. I'm not going anywhere. I love you. I'm going to do everything I can to make sure that I'll be here for you,' I said, but he really didn't know how to act.

"I could tell he was upset and bothered by it, but he's thirteen, and boys aren't supposed to cry. So he took it like a man and did the best that he could do. It got to the point that he didn't want me talking about it at all, and he'd even get mad at me if I did. When I shaved my hair, my husband and I were on the back porch and I said, 'Here's your one chance to cut Mama's hair.' But he wouldn't even come out.

"It was so hard. My doctors made me feel like I was not worth anything. I was laying there exposed, with them poking me, and they wouldn't even let me ask them

"**I got** fifty dollars to be a fake patient who the residents tried to figure out what was wrong with me. I had to keep quiet but I kept wanting to tell them they were asking me everything but the one right question. They hadn't a clue."

—*Krista Hale, 39*

questions. My oncologist put his finger to his lips, telling me to be quiet. They acted like I was so stupid and low that I was not worthy of asking about my own health. It was humiliating. I may not be in the medical field, I may not be the smartest person in the world, but it is my body, and I got a right to know what's going to happen to me when you take a muscle from my back to recreate a breast. When I asked my doctor how bad chemo was, he said, 'If it was so bad, everybody would not be doing it.'

"I found great comfort in the Bible. I wouldn't get out of the car at the hospital without first reading some verses. I liked Psalm 23 the best and pictured the verse while they were giving me chemo. I could visualize myself by the still waters in the green pastures. When the nurse was giving me the chemo that's called Red Devil, I'd think, I fear no evil. He is leading me in the path of righteousness.

"**I watched** a lot of VH1 shows about the fabulous life of so-and-so and I'd think: you don't have cancer. I'd look at regular people on the street and think you don't have to do this and I do. Not like my life is so bad, I just feel so different from everyone else."

—*Melissa Sorenson, 25*

"I know what medicine and doctors can do for you, but I ultimately feel God is in control. If I did not have faith in God, I do not think I would be here. I could just feel myself going downhill with depression and terrible anxiety. I got afraid to even go out of the house. I started to not enjoy being around people. I felt so ugly and ashamed with no hair. I was so sick, I felt like I had fire shooting out of my head, and I was throwing up so much. They kept telling me, 'You shouldn't be this sick. You are not responding like other people.'"

As Tracy spoke, I flashed back to a day during my own treatment. Sitting statuesque at my kitchen table in front of a plate of iodine-free spaghetti, I could not make my hands work. The familiar function of curling my fingers around a fork was impossible. I asked my doctors about the temporary paralysis in my arms and legs and the severe waves of fatigue that rendered me unable to speak. Underwhelmed with concern, they muttered, 'Most people in your condition are still able to go to work.' Tracy, Seth, and many other patients I met received similar retorts from their doctors: 'In thirty years of practice I've never seen anyone as sensitive to treatment as you.' 'You are just not behaving the way most patients do.'

Why had the patients I met elicited such similar responses from our doctors? Perhaps the young adult cancer patients whose bodies played by the rules were at the gym, a frat party, or their kids' soccer games, instead of revisiting their cancer into my voice recorder. Or maybe we, the hypersensitive outlier patients, are more of the twenty- and thirtysomething norm than our doctors recognize. Out of 13,000 practicing oncologists in the United States, a scant handful focus exclusively on young adult oncology. The majority of our doctors have zero expertise with the physiology of young adult cancer patients. Perhaps our doctors never see anyone who reacts like us because they just don't see many patients in our age range. If clinical trials for our treatment regimens are conducted on graying baby boomers instead of on young adults, why would doctors expect us to respond as the rest of their patients do?

Tracy continued her story of being told she was outside the norm. "I would just be at home, standing and looking out the window, thinking everybody else is going on with their life, going to work, going to school, and I can't do nothing. Sometimes I couldn't hardly get out of bed or take a shower because I was so tired. It upset me so bad when I thought about my son. My mind was so foggy that he had to wear his braces longer than he needed to because I forgot to take him to the orthodontist. There were plenty of times when I drove just five minutes up the road, and I'd have to stop and lay down in the car. I didn't tell people, though. My husband is a very loving, caring, supportive person. He's also very protective. He wants to be in control, and when I was feeling this bad, it's like he had no control. All he could do was go to chemo with me, rub my back, help me get dressed or take a bath.

"**We give** way more license for pets to lay around the house and rest after surgery than we do for people. I wanted to take time for myself but it felt too indulgent, like I was supposed to just keep on going."

—*Debbie Ng, 27*

"My family and doctors are saying you need to get out and exercise, but they just didn't understand how extremely sick I was. I pressed for new medication to help with the side effects. My doctor was out of town so the nurse asked a different doctor for the prescription. When I picked it up from their office, the nurse said to me in front of all the other patients, 'The doctor said for you to be as sick as you are, it must have spread to your brain and everywhere else.' I said, 'Well, thank you, you just told me I'm dying.'

"I was in disbelief at her carelessness. I had these little voices perched on each shoulder. One is saying, 'You ain't got nothing to worry about. It's all right. My doctor would have told me if he found out it spread.' But the voice on the other shoulder is saying, 'The nurse told you it has already spread everywhere. You're dead meat.'

"I don't believe in suicide. Religion says it's wrong, and even if you're not religious, it's not a good thing to do for the people that you leave behind who care about you and have to live wondering if there was something they could have done. But still, I remember thinking, What's the use? I've got several more chemo treatments left. I got radiation. I got to take Tamoxifen for five years. They are pumping all this crap into me and don't know what it will do to my body down the line. So when I walked out of that doctor's office, I did think about killing myself 'cause she told me I was dying. Why let my family, my thirteen-year-old son watch me suffer and die? I could have easily run my car off the road. It would look like an accident, and nobody would've known.

> "**I could not** stand to look at my shaved head. I took baths for eight months because of my catheter and made my mom put a washcloth over the waterspout so I couldn't see my reflection in it."
>
> —Dana Merk, 24

"Being sick, no hair, and throwing up all the time, can't eat, can't sleep for days even with sleeping pills, people telling you you're dying. All this kind of stuff compounded together knocked me down about as low as you can get. I think my husband and several other people started feeling kind of put out with me. For a period of time, they're all taking care of you and doing everything for you, but at some point you're kind of like a burden. Or they get tired of coming home to you being sick. I can imagine that's bad, but there ain't nothing I can do about it.

"I was here by myself looking in the mirror or out the window, just getting depressed. I'm not even talking to anybody. Partly, I didn't want them to worry, but at the same time I was thinking, If I tell them that I'm feeling like this, they'd say, 'You've got something wrong mentally. You need to be on medicine, you need to see a psychologist.' I had fear that they were going to tell me again, 'You're not a strong person. You're not handling this the way that you should be.'

"I seriously think chemo affects your brain, it affects your body. I was not in a normal state of mind. I don't know if other people experience that, but I was not thinking logically. One day I was home alone, so very sick, I couldn't eat or be with my family or do anything, couldn't get up out of bed. I was in such extreme pain. I thought, My quality of life just sucks, so I don't care what kind of quantity I have. I have no quality, and nobody around me does, either, because they have to take care of me. They have to clean the house and cook supper 'cause I can't do anything. I felt like a worthless piece of crap. I've got a gun. And just for an instant, I thought of that gun and I thought . . . Now, in my normal mind state, I would never sit there and think about this. It would destroy my son, my husband. I could never do anything like that. But at that time I was hurting so bad and it was so intense that I just thought, It's never going to get any better. I am never going to get over this. Everybody around me is suffering, I can't do it anymore. I literally started giving up. That may sound stupid, because compared to what a lot of other people go through, I could have had it a lot worse, but the effects of the drugs on my body, and the way doctors made me feel like a number, a statistic, a chart. I got to the point where I didn't even care anymore.

"I got in my car and went to the church. I talked to Brother Leon, a pastor in his seventies, and I told him what was going on with me. He gave me Bible verses, and we talked. I asked if we could go to the altar together. I got down on my knees and put my hands up. I was so weak and sick, I thought I was going to pass out. I said,

"**I don't have** anything in my heart anymore. I can't cry. Can't feel anything anymore because I've let it go and go and go and there is a stopping place somewhere."

—*Krista Hale, 39*

'I don't know where to start or what to say.' Brother Leon told me, 'Just say whatever is in your heart.' I started crying. I had been so strong, I had not cried since my diagnosis because I thought that moping and carrying on would be seen as a weakness. I was crying and crying and crying, and Brother Leon started crying with me. Brother Leon told me, 'Just say what is in your heart.'

"When I finally got composure, I said, 'God, please give me peace. All I want or need is peace to accept my fate, whether I survive or whether I don't. Thank you for letting it be me because I wouldn't want it to be anybody else.' I couldn't handle it if it was my child—I mean, I would if I had to. I asked God for peace, but I did not ask to be cured. I felt like that would be selfish. If it was time for me to go, I think I had in a way already accepted it. It's not that I don't think He can cure me, because I think He can. But I feel like He has a destiny for me, and if that is for me to die of breast cancer, then I will suck it up and do the best I can.

"For me to sit here and accept what I have been through and be able to talk about it, deal with it, not hide it, not be ashamed, I think it makes me a strong person. I think it shows character. There are a lot of women who can say they went through cancer and didn't get depressed, didn't have anxiety, didn't cry. They still jogged their five miles a day and were a normal person. That's not me. I am a normal person that went through a terrible, horrible experience.

"I eventually realized it might be good for me to go to the young survivor breast cancer group and was excited to meet new friends who could relate to what I had been through. Everybody there was like a sassy wonder woman, ready to go beat somebody's butt, like 'I am a cancer survivor, hear me roar.' I'm not sassy. I'm just a person, a human being. I am strong and I survived, but cancer was really bad. Nobody was talking about the hard things, like complaints with the hospital or doctors or what it was like to experience not feeling good. Unless you had something positive to say, they didn't want to hear it. It made me wonder if something was wrong with me. I don't think there is, but I was the only person who showed any sign of weakness.

> **"A lot of** people try to build you up emotionally with false cheeriness. I just want someone to say, 'This really, really sucks.'"
>
> —*Jill Woods, 38*

"Where do you find people who can be honest and true with themselves about this experience? Some people think that after an experience like cancer, if you are not smiling and doing cartwheels every day, then you're just sitting around and feeling sorry for yourself. I am grateful to be alive, but I have good days and bad days just like I did before cancer. I also believe you can't help yourself if you deny that you have suffered. I felt sad when I walked out of that meeting. I came home to my house, which has pink ribbon symbols everywhere, and it just made me feel like I was in a sisterhood or a sorority that I didn't ask to be in, and I feel like I don't belong because I don't act like I'm supposed to."

Tracy's disappointment with the cancer community—even with the young adult community—surprised me. I was an East Coast liberal Jew, born to kvetch and form contrary opinions. I had staged sit-ins in my high school cafeteria and stormed board meetings at Columbia University. Where there was an institution, I wanted to crush it. Tracy, however, seemed like a nonconfrontational joiner who was at home with being part of an establishment. Yet even she, who plastered her house with pink ribbons, felt alienated by a cancer community that transformed her hardship into a cheerleading cry.

Tracy continued, "I finally started seeing a therapist and got onto medication. I wish I could talk to people who were just diagnosed and say, 'If you need help, it is okay. If you need to take Zoloft because you are having a problem, it doesn't mean that you are mental or are going to be put away. It means that you have been diagnosed with a serious, potentially deadly disease, and that is hard.' I don't want anybody else walking to their car from the doctor's office thinking, I'm going to die so maybe I should end it now.

"Through my therapist, I became the patient advocate on the Distress Management Team at my hospital. It is made up of doctors, nurses, social workers, and chaplains. Our goal is to design ways to help patients deal with the stress of cancer. When I was diagnosed, all my doctors did was tell me to try to be in a good mood and watch funny movies. I should not have had to get as low as I got before somebody finally helped me, and it took me months and months to drag myself back up.

> "Hard times bring some couples together. Not us. My divorce date was exactly three hundred sixty-five days from my diagnosis."
>
> —Katie Smith, 37

"My son, my husband, my whole family pretty much, they've all gotten to a point where they don't like me talking about cancer. They have no interest in it and don't want to hear it. They think it's better for me not to talk about it or be involved in it. It's hard. I feel like I have nobody supporting me, nobody backing me. Everyone is telling me to move beyond it, which makes me feel stupid. I think there are other people out there like me who feel alone, who want to be real and talk about what is going on with them after such an experience.

"Me, my husband, and my son, we lost a certain kind of innocence. Before you get sick, you are almost living in a fairy-tale world and don't really notice the bad stuff. Then all of a sudden you get sick and it's all you notice. It's like something was taken away that you can't ever get back again. There is a lot of continued worry that I have to deal with, even after the people around me have gotten back to their normal lives. I still have long-term side effects. At some point my breast is going to have to be reconstructed. I am still seeing four doctors on a regular basis. I wish I could put it behind me, but I can't.

"I'm turning forty soon, and I know everyone will say, 'Lordy, lordy, Tracy's turning forty.' But I thank the Lord for letting me be here. There is no better thing to me than being able to watch my son grow up and just live life."

On our way out to her garage we ducked into the basement TV room, which was filled wall to wall with Harley Davidson paraphernalia. Tracy's son and husband had come home and were sitting with the dog watching TV. As soon as I stepped into the room, I had the feeling of crossing into enemy territory. Tracy's husband went through the motions of introducing himself but kept his attention on the TV. I felt like a social worker on an unwanted home visit and couldn't wait to leave.

At the end of our twelve-hour day together, Tracy drove me to my hotel and got me settled in my room. Before leaving, she said, "You are so brave. I can't imagine traveling alone to a city I've never been to and don't know a soul. I'm gonna call and check in on you, and you call me if you need anything at all. Know you are always welcome at my house." I thanked Tracy for her kindness but shrugged off her amazement at my bravery. I explained that in my early and mid-twenties, I had traveled alone in Indonesia, drove cross-country by myself, and camped alone in the mountains of Utah. Four days in Birmingham with friendly cancer patients was easy.

After she left, I crawled into bed feeling spent and inexplicably nervous about my meetings scheduled for the next few days. Many people say that cancer has transformed them into audacious, adventurous risk takers. With Tracy's offer echoing in my head, I realized how increasingly hesitant and afraid a person I had become since my diagnosis. The days I had boasted about, of solo jet-setting, suddenly felt like many decades ago.

Perhaps it was seeing how delicate life is or how easily things can go awry that caused me to feel this way. As much as it surprised me to admit it, I was glad that Tracy was nearby, just in case I felt the unlikely and unforeseeable need to call.

RESOURCES

Emotional Support

Existential funks, nail biting, and temper tantrums in the privacy of my apartment were the bedrock moments of my cancer experience. On some days, smashing raw eggs against my shower wall alleviated my angst or depression, but other days called for a more hard-core introspective approach to surmounting the emotional ambush of cancer.

Feeling sad, blue, angry, and overwhelmed are normal, appropriate responses to cancer and do not mean that you have depression or anxiety.

But if you feel that these normal emotions are spinning beyond your control, are making you extremely distraught, or last for a prolonged time, follow Tracy's lead and talk to your doctor or a social worker about being evaluated for depression or anxiety.

The Facts

- About 25 percent of all cancer patients suffer from clinical depression.
- Young adult cancer patients have an increased risk of developing depression, anxiety, and post-traumatic stress disorder.
- Contrary to popular opinion, large clinical trials (most notably, the Emotional Well-Being Study conducted in 2007 at the University of Pennsylvania, with more than a thousand patients) have proved that emotions are not linked to cancer outcomes.

■ Although depression, anxiety, and other "negative" thoughts will not cause your cancer to grow or hasten your death, they do make for a poor quality of life and should be addressed.

The Experts

The licensed social workers at CancerCare and the Ulman Cancer Fund for Young Adults excel in meeting the needs of young adults. Through over-the-phone counseling, they will help you strategize around your practical and emotional needs and will assist in identifying a good therapist in your area, should you want one. Visit CancerCare, www.cancercare.org, 800-813-HOPE (4673); and the Ulman Cancer Fund for Young Adults, ulmanfund.org, 888-393-FUND (3863).

No One Is an Island

Cancer patients who experience isolation are more prone to depression. Check out Peer Support on page 100 to find myriad ways to connect to other young adults with cancer.

Coping with Pain

Are you terrified of becoming a morphine addict, screaming down the halls for the nurse to give you your next fix? When I talked with Dr. Diane Meier, the director of the Center to Advance Palliative Care, she debunked the myths of pain management and talked about ways that twenty- and thirtysomething patients can stand up for our rights to improve the quality of our lives with less pain and less stress.

Five Myths about Pain Management and Pain Meds

If I take morphine and other opioid pain meds, I'll become addicted.

Wrong. An extremely small segment of patients become addicted. Addiction is a psychiatric illness that exists in the patient prior to a diagnosis or the use of pain medication.

Pain management meds are for people who are near death.

Wrong. Pain management can be used at all stages of illness and can help with side effects such as fatigue, insomnia, constipation, nausea, dry mouth, and mouth sores.

If I ask for pain management, that means I'm not fighting hard enough.

Wrong. Managing your pain can greatly improve the quality of your life, allow you to participate in more activities, and be more social. People with untreated pain are more likely to die sooner, so receiving pain management is a part of good medical care.

I won't benefit from a pain-management team because I already have an oncologist and nurses.

Wrong. Prescribing and monitoring pain medication is the exclusive focus of a palliative care team or another pain-management specialist. They often understand better than an oncologist or an oncology nurse the nuances of these medications and how to minimize the side effects of opioid drugs.

If I take pain meds now, they won't be effective later and I'll have no backup.

Wrong. Palliative care or other pain-management specialists know how to prescribe and dose medications that can give effective relief for different symptoms at different phases of your care.

What Is Palliative Care and How Can I Get It?

- *Palliative care*, also known as supportive care, focuses on relieving pain and other symptoms associated with serious illness.

Care is often given by an interdisciplinary team consisting of a doctor, a nurse, and a social worker.

- It is easy to confuse hospice with palliative care, but they are different. Hospice is for the patient who is dying and no longer receiving treatment. Palliative care is given at any phase of your illness and while you are still actively taking treatment.

- Don't let anyone trivialize your pain. You have a right to ask for, and even demand, pain treatment. Tell your doctor or nurse that you would like to meet with a palliative care team or a pain-management expert.

- Visit the Web site of the Center to Advance Palliative Care, www.getpalliativecare.org, to learn more about palliative care and insurance, check out quick facts, determine whether palliative care is right for you, and read patients' stories.

- Find a palliative care team in your area. Search the "Provider Directory" at Getpalliativecare.org. If a palliative care expert is not available through a hospital, check with a hospice in your area to see whether it delivers nonhospice palliative care.

9

It Girl

In my five years as a cancer consumer, I had encountered mostly cold and impersonal hospital staff who used our national healthcare crisis as a poor excuse for treating patients like plastic tchotchkes on an assembly line in China. On day two of my Alabama trip, UAB staff members, including the executive director of the Comprehensive Cancer Center, met with me individually and spoke about their interests in providing supportive care for young adult patients. Absent was the I'm-too-busy-for-anything-but-the-bottom-line attitude. Maybe it was just Southern hospitality onstage in a hospital; regardless of the reason, I now had proof that congeniality is possible in an American medical institution.

The cancer center reserved a conference room for me, where, over the next three days, I could meet one-on-one with young adult patients who drove in from surrounding small cities and tiny towns. Mary Ann Harvard and I sat among eight empty high-backed swivel chairs at a long oval conference table—a sleek contrast to my other recorded conversations, which took place in dilapidated art studios or on Dumpster-dive couches. In dress slacks and heels and wielding a pad of notes with high-lighted excerpts from her journal, Mary Ann looked like a hybrid of a young college student and the White House press secretary. I expected her to speak in sound bites. Instead, her words were genuine and profound as she detailed the private and monumental life issues she was facing.

"I think when you are young and female, you are less likely to be diagnosed than anyone else. I know that from my own experience. I was twenty-two, and my doctors thought I didn't have anything wrong with me. I was labeled anorexic because of my weight loss. One asthma doctor even wrote on a little prescription form: 'Needs to see psychiatrist.' The cancer was controlling my life. I couldn't walk upstairs or talk on the phone because of the constant cough. This had been going on for two and a half years. I was seeing doctors once or twice a week before my diagnosis, but they just saw me as a hypochondriac.

"My mother finally got me to a doctor who did a chest X-ray and blood work, and she had a look on her face like, 'You should be dead right now.' I checked into the hospital that night. My husband, Mark, who was then my fiancé, was in the room with me when the doctor sat on my bed and said, 'You have cancer.' I immediately cried and cried and cried, and then I picked my head up and said, 'Thank you, God. Finally, finally, someone has figured out what is wrong with me.' I wasn't sad. I was relieved.

"Hodgkin's lymphoma is highly curable if it's caught early, but my tumor was the size of a football and occupied my whole chest. It moved my heart and my lungs so I was only breathing at 25 percent capacity. I don't know how I had managed to work part-time at the Hallmark store and be a full-time student with cancer that was so advanced. My oncologist said I had a fifty-fifty chance of complete remission.

"My general practitioner had failed to watch a spot on my chest X-ray that he saw two and a half years earlier. Lots of people have told me they would have sued him. Well, all the money in the world isn't gonna take away what's happened. It wasn't gonna make me well. I'm angry in a lot of different ways. I'm angry at him, and I'm angry at every doctor who ignored me. In the back of my mind I regret not going to the emergency room, but I had said to myself earlier, Why do I need to go to the emergency room if I'm going to all of these doctors? I feel in my heart that I did everything that I could've done, and I hope it wasn't because of my age and gender that I got what seems like unequal treatment.

"My mother's goal in life is to figure out what caused my cancer. She'll go into detective mode: 'I think it was caused by that breakup with your ex-boyfriend when you were so extremely upset.' I say, 'Momma, if we knew what caused cancer, we would have a cure for it.' I would love to have prevented whatever caused this, but I try to meditate and think that this has happened and all I can do now is choose how to react to it. But I do wonder sometimes, Did I cause my cancer? Did I let this happen to me?"

As these words tumbled out of Mary Ann's mouth, I wanted to hug and slap her in a single grand gesture. In half an hour of knowing Mary Ann, I felt an affection that made me want to defend her the way I would my brother or my cousins. If one can experience love at first sight with a partner, I could only assume that love at first sight can happen with a friendship, too. Mary Ann's honesty, gutsiness, and questioning of authority were void of the badass, fuck-cancer, leftover teenage angst that gripped much of the young adult cancer community, and which I, too, often possessed. Though only twenty-six years old, Mary Ann seemed wiser and more dignified than people three times her age and I wanted to save her maturity from the base-less thinking that our emotions can cause our cancer.

Mary Ann's comments about causing her own cancer evoked in me memories of my own diagnosis when the Louise Hay crazies crawled out of the woodwork, explaining that I had caused my own cancer as a result of my inability to express myself. I responded to these well-meaning accusers with a caustic, bordering on vulgar, self-defense, and they quickly learned that I have had zero problem with self-expression. Over time, I added to my arsenal of retorts a list of clinical studies disproving archaic theories that patients' emotions cause our horrific diseases. If simply expressing our emotions was a viable method of cancer prevention, I'd be overjoyed to never have a pap smear or a breast exam again, and I could check colonoscopies off my "after fifty" to-do list; the government would have justifica-tion for its decreases in National Cancer Institute funding; and my inbox would not be clogged with pledge forms from women in pink walking for the cure. I restrained myself with Mary Ann and told her that if a broken heart caused cancer, I don't know a woman in the world who would not have been diagnosed by her mid-twenties.

Mary Ann agreed and continued to talk about her life as a college student. "I needed to be enrolled in college in order to stay on my parents' health insurance, so I had to go to school all through treat-ment. I didn't want to go; I had to go. It's difficult getting chemo on Friday and being back at school on Tuesday. Everyone else was in a sorority or occupied with studying full-time. I felt left out, like I didn't belong a lot. I wish students and teachers would have been more wel-coming to me. Most of my teachers didn't care about my condition, except for my history teacher. I was like her child, and it hurt her to see me going through so much pain. She was extremely understanding and let me enroll in her classes with an automatic withdrawal so I could go to school part-time and still get insurance. When I turned twenty-five, I got kicked off of my parents' health insurance. Mark and I knew we'd have to get married for insurance, even if it was just a courthouse wedding. We had been engaged for quite a while and were happy to get married anyway.

"Sometimes I'll tell Mark, 'Do you realize that you've never known me when I was well?' I've felt sick the entire time I've known him. When we were dating, I would have to cut the evening short or cancel plans, and he made these accommodations to help me, not even knowing what was wrong with me. I hear about women with cancer whose husbands leave them. Mark was just my fiancé. All he gave me was a ring; he wasn't obligated. I have never worried about Mark leaving me. He didn't leave when he could have, so I just knew that he was always gonna be here for me. He is definitely amazing. Mark understands how I'm feeling better than anyone. Other people are overly positive, saying, 'You'll be fine, you'll get through it.' But when I don't feel good, I want someone to feel sorry for me sometimes or understand that this is really hard.

"Mark has always been my advocate. When the lab technicians are digging around for a vein, he says to them, 'If I hear her so much as whimper, we are calling this off.' It hurts so bad when they stick your hand, it's like they've just done the Jesus to you. Sometimes I have to step outside and detach myself from my body because it helps me handle the pain better. In my head, I tell them, 'It's just my body, do what you have to do.' It's just my arm, it is not my soul. If I give them my body, it is easier than having them take it. If I put my arm out and say, 'Just do it,' it is like they are not forcing me, and the pain sometimes is not as difficult. Sometimes I'll just say some Hail Marys and Our Fathers, and the pain will pass. Sometimes it is hard to do that. Pain is pain. It's real. It hurts.

"**I always** envisioned how I'd look as a bride, and bald and fat weren't in the picture. Most brides worry about whether to wear their hair up or down, not if they have enough hair and how to clip the fake hair to their head."

—*Jill Woods, 38*

"**If I had** a baby, it would probably glow in the dark after what I've been through. I joke, but not having a kid is my one regret about cancer. I doubt I'll ever be able to adopt because of the condition I've had, but I'd love to adopt a thrown away or tormented child and love it like it was my own."

—*Krista Hale, 39*

"Mark and I got married this year when I was cancer-free, and then eight months later my cancer came back. I was really, really mad. I said, 'Why, God, would you let me get married and show me what it is like to live a semi-normal life and then take that away?' I find it hard to look at my wedding pictures because it wasn't just my wedding, it was a day to celebrate what Mark and I had overcome together. It is hard to look back at those eight months and think, Did I live as much as I could? I try to accept what has been given to me, but it is not easy.

"Mark wakes up at 2 A.M. for his job at the radio station, and in the afternoon he edits wedding videos at home. He works two, sometimes three jobs. He'll fall asleep driving or in the shower, but he keeps going 'cause he knows what has to be done. He sleeps less, just to spend time with me. We like being at home together because it's private. I lived with my parents until our wedding so we are still getting used to our married life. Mark makes fun of me 'cause one of my favorite little hobbies is reading the grocery store ads and finding the cheapest price. It is like a game to me, trying to save as much as I can. We don't have trouble paying bills, but we don't have extra, especially if we eventually adopt a child.

"More than likely, I cannot have children from the treatments and transplant. We don't even want to try because there are so many ifs. I haven't had a menstrual cycle in a year and a half. I don't feel like I'm female, I feel like an it. I have a hard time seeing people with their babies. I'm not mad at them that they can have a baby, but it makes it real for me that I can't. Of course, Mark is understanding, and I am so thankful he is, but sometimes I tell him, 'This is not easy, even though you are okay with it.' This is something nobody can fix, and I feel robbed because I know what my cancer has taken away from me.

"From my head to toes, I have been affected by cancer. Every part of my body has changed. I don't feel sexy or female. I feel mutilated. I feel different. I can't fix my hair, and wearing a wig just feels like a cover-up so people don't stare. I don't feel beautiful, and that is hard, especially when you are married. Mark will say, 'I love you just the way you are.' It is comforting for him to be easygoing, but I don't feel attractive. Feeling attractive goes into and is combined with feeling sexy, which might put you in the mood.

"Cancer is hard** on your sex life. I don't want to be touched. I'm touched all day and have no sense of what my body is anymore. It belongs to the doctors."

—Amilca Mouton-Fuentes, 26

Usually, I don't feel like I'm in that mood. When you have been married for nine months, people think you are making love every night. It feels like something is missing to not be able to or want to do that. I feel like I am cheating Mark a little bit because it's part of marriage. It doesn't cause arguments, he doesn't get mad, but I feel like I can't be there for him like I should. I think it affects me more than it affects him. I feel like we should be engaged in it all the time, and we are not.

"Mark deals with his frustration and stress through humor and jokes. He says he and his friends don't talk about serious stuff so it just builds up and it eats him alive. Most people are overly optimistic with him: 'Oh, she'll just pull through this. Y'all are going to be fine.' That is not realistic. Sometimes you just want someone to listen to you.

"As difficult as my transplant was for me, it was that difficult for him. He'd sleep, do his laundry, and take a shower on the bone marrow transplant unit. When he'd leave the hospital for work at 2 A.M., he'd go to the parking deck and sit in the car and just beat the steering wheel and scream and cry at the top of his lungs. Sometimes I'll hide my feelings in order to help him because it is so difficult for him. It is not fair that he has to go through this, too. I try to talk to him about it, but he usually says his feelings don't matter or he doesn't have time to deal with the way that he feels.

"Two nights ago, I tried to tell Mark I feel like my death is soon. It upset him, but I'm like, 'I want to tell you—I have to tell somebody. And I'm not saying I want you to believe me, but I want you to hear me out and understand that these feelings are real.' I told Mark I don't want my coffin opened. My close family can see me, but I don't want others staring at me, going, 'Oh—don't she look good?' I tell myself I can't do anything to prevent it or change it, it's just gonna happen when it's gonna happen. But I hope it's not soon. I would hope God would not do that to me or to my family, especially since Mark and I have been married for such a short time. I have a scan coming up soon, and I think, What am I gonna hear? Did my treatment work? It's scary, and it is hard to talk about with other people. I was so close to dying the first time, and I wonder why I didn't. Sometimes I wish that I had died, rather than have to keep getting well, getting sick, getting well, getting sick.

"I wonder if heaven is different things to different people, instead of one big place that everyone goes to. Mark thinks heaven is the most wonderful place you can imagine and hell is the worst place that you can imagine. If you have a fear of heights, then you're just hanging off a building every day. To me, that kinda makes sense. I would think of heaven as Dr Pepper and Reese's cups, M&M cookies and going to the spa to get my hair and nails done every day. I wonder if you can float around invisible on the earth after you die? Could I go visit Mark? Would I have that ability to be an angel?

"I don't know if it's possible for someone to know when the end is near. I don't know if I'm just making it up or if I actually know. It is so real to me that it is terrifying to feel like I know something so serious. I don't even know who to approach with those feelings. If I know I'm gonna die soon, is there something I'm supposed to do before I die? I have never flown on an airplane before or gone places, and it would be nice to do that, but more than wanting to do that, I just want to be who I am, to live my life being honest, not hurting anyone. That kinda thing. I do feel like I'm not gonna live much longer, and Mark is the only person that I've really said that to. I don't feel like he believes me, or maybe he doesn't wanna believe it himself.

"I don't want to live if I don't have a good quality of life, if I can't function, feed myself, use the bathroom. That's not only hard on me, but it's hard on everyone around me. I would never attempt to take my own life, but I don't want to be kept alive on life support. A living will has crossed my mind, but I haven't acted on it. In my situation, that's probably something that would be good to do. Even though my family and I are Catholic, I think they would accept that.

"One afternoon at the clinic, I was so angry and frustrated I wanted to give up. I sat on the hallway floor, leaning against the wall, just crying and not caring who saw me. Out of nowhere, a woman with terminal breast cancer asked if she could sit down next to me, and we talked. She was literally an angel sent to me at the lowest point in my life. She was so positive, but it wasn't a fake positive. She knew how to make the best out of the worst situation and showed me what matters is your quality of life, not how long you live. A positive attitude is not going to cure me, but it will help me have a better quality of life. This doesn't mean I'm always feeling positive. It is more of a willingness to accept the way that I feel, rather than thinking I have to be strong. If I'm sad or depressed, I allow myself to feel it. I try to let something positive come out of this awful experience, but it is not always going to feel positive along the way.

"When you have a disease like cancer, who you are changes and you have to find out who you've become and what you are supposed to do. Before cancer, I had my goals and I knew how to achieve them. I wanted to finish college and become a first-grade teacher. I was so passionate about it and only had a year and a half left of school. Now I'm not sure of things like I was before. It is hard to not be sure. Knowing what is going to happen brings me comfort. At the end of last semester, I prayed so hard and asked, Am I supposed to go back to school? I wonder if being diagnosed the second time was the Lord's way of saying that I should not go back. I don't feel like my heart is there. Right smack in my college career, I learned maybe college is not what I want after all.

"Mark and I play the question game. I ask him a question, then he asks me a question. I asked him, 'Mark, what do you see me doing?' He said, 'I see you being a lobbyist.' I've always wanted a reason to own business suits. I don't know why. I cruise through the department store, and I want those business suits that are 'dry clean only.' Maybe the business suit symbolizes power because I want people to hear me. This little part of me that is a fighter can get fired up and loud and aggressive. I want people to respect me and go, 'She knows what she's talking about.'

"I have never been an outgoing person, but now I don't hide a lot anymore. I was asked to speak about my cancer experience to a support group last week. When I walked in the front door after talking to that support group, Mark said, 'You are so happy, whatever you did, I want you to do it every day.' When I was talking to those people, their faces were glued to me. If I turned my head, they turned their heads. I didn't know I was capable of capturing people's attention."

Lying in bed that night in my quiet hotel room, I thought about Mary Ann. She was high on the list of powerful women I had met in my lifetime, but she wore her provocative and incendiary attitude in her back pocket, rather than on her sleeve, like so many of us. She explained intense feelings and experiences in lucid, unexaggerated terms. Her lack of charisma was surprisingly exquisite and commanding. Only a few times in my life had I met people who expressed themselves so simply yet profoundly. Mary Ann was one of these enigmatic people. I knew I wanted her in my life far into the future.

RESOURCES

Young Adult Caregivers

Every year, there are an estimated 30,000 new young adult cancer spouses in the United States. This figure does not include domestic partners or dating relationships. These are the people who learn by trial and error how to wash our hair in the kitchen sink, change our bandages, and chew out the scheduling nurse, while holding down a full-time job and paying the bills.

Most young adult caregivers narrow their social lives, reduce the time they spend with their families, and often sacrifice educational opportunities and activities that would lead to career advancement. "Partners of Cancer Survivors at Risk for Depression," a study published in the *Journal of Clinical Oncology* in 2007, showed that partners and survivors suffer from similar quality-of-life and mental health issues. Unfortunately, partners were less likely to receive treatment for these conditions and reported less spiritual well-being, less marital satisfaction, and a greater feeling of loneliness than survivors did. Taking care of another without taking care of yourself is clearly detrimental to your own health.

Help the Helper

Young Cancer Spouses, www.youngcancerspouses.org. This sleek Web site is a gold mine of detailed information for young adult caregivers, regardless of marital status. Its high-traffic, password-protected bulletin board is a safe space for spouses and partners to vent. No patients allowed!

CancerCare, www.cancercare.org, 800-813-HOPE (4673). This organization offers telephone, online, and in-person (New York area) support groups for young adult caregivers.

Strength for Caring, www.strengthforcaring.com, 888-ICARE80 (888-422-7380). The "Caregiver Manual" and "Daily Care" sections of this Web site are excellent 101 crash courses for first-time caregivers.

Well Spouse Association, www.wellspouse.org, 800-838-0879. This organization provides one-on-one mentoring with a seasoned caregiver who may be older than his or her twenties and thirties but has loads of experience to coach you along the way.

Build Support

You are not Superman or Superwoman. You cannot do everything yourself. Read Building Support Systems on page 115, and put a friend in charge of activating your community to help you.

Five Insights on Caregiving

The following tips for caregivers are from Matt Herynk, the founding director of YoungCancerSpouses.

1. The best time saver: have a friend post updates on a blog to cut down on your needing to return phone calls.

2. What you wish you had done sooner: take time for yourself. You have to, because if you fall apart, everything else falls apart.

3. The hardest part: trying to keep it all running.

4. The worst part: watching your partner suffer, knowing there's absolutely nothing you can do about it.

5. The rewards: we became closer, more intimate, but not in ways we would ever have wanted to, given the choice.

Student Life

Can you keep up with your friends at a bar, eat your super-green cancer diet in the dining hall, hide your scars in a shared bathroom, and fight off each wave of strep throat rippling through your dorm? Are your friends concerned with papers, grades, and Greek life, while you are focused on just saving your life? Does your major feel meaningless after you have stared death in the face? Do you wonder whether you can even afford to finish college or trade school? Is your health insurance in jeopardy each time you jump from part-time, to full-time, to leave of absence?

Those in the Know

The Ulman Cancer Fund for Young Adults, www.ulmanfund.org, 888-393-FUND (3863). Take advantage of its scholarships and over-the-phone social workers who can help you navigate the challenges of surviving cancer and student life.

Carolyn's Compassionate Children, www.cccscholarships.org, 866-540-1392. Visit CCC's stellar database of 3,000 scholarships for higher education. Their blog includes webinars and tips on surviving college with cancer.

The SAM Fund for Young Adult Survivors of Cancer, www .thesamfund.org. This organization provides scholarships and grants to college, grad, and vocational students for entrance exam fees, application fees, school interview travel expenses, utilities, gym memberships, and more.

Five Tips on Getting Scholarships and Grants

When you are competing against other cancer patients for limited scholarship funds, just using the "cancer card" is not enough. Give yourself an edge by following these suggestions from Samantha Eisenstein, the founder and director of the SAM Fund:

1. Read the application thoroughly to make sure you qualify; call the organization for clarification.

2. Answer all questions with complete and direct responses.

3. Write your best.

4. Have at least one other person edit your application.

5. Double-check to make sure you have included any necessary supporting documents.

Best Secret for Surviving School

Even if you do not want to, or think you do not need to, always tell a school counselor and all of your teachers about your cancer at the start of each semester or as soon as you are diagnosed. Ask how and when to request assignment extensions and build extra time into your own calender to meet deadlines.

Five Steps to Staying Well in School

Communal living is a germ fest. Take reasonable precautions to stay well.

1. Ask your doctor if you should get a flu shot.

2. Use hand sanitizer religiously. Do not touch your face without sanitizing your hands.

3. Clean computer keyboards that others have touched.

4. Do not share utensils, drinking glasses, makeup, or eye or nasal drops.

5. Buy new toothbrushes and launder washcloths frequently; store them separately from your roommates'.

10

The Fix

I had four hours before my plane left Birmingham in which to meet with Greg Dawson. The cancer center was closed on a Saturday morning, so I scouted out a quiet corner of the lobby outside of my hotel's grand ballroom. Five minutes into our conversation, we were interrupted by a flotilla of housekeeping women with shrieking industrial vacuum cleaners. I was pressed for time, and although I knew it was stupid to head up to my hotel room with a perfect stranger (after all, cancer patients can be rapists and axe murderers, too), I did it anyway.

With most other patients, I had a good fifteen minutes of casual conversation to break the ice before I pressed the record button. Not so with Greg. He was a straightforward, edgy storyteller, who immediately plunged into the meat of the matter. A thirty-six-year-old

> **"You have** to try hard. Cancer isn't something you can do halfway."
>
> —Krista Hale, 39

engineer diagnosed with thymoma at age twenty-seven, Greg had a recurrence at thirty-one that necessitated the removal of one lung.

"I had an intensity to bite the heads off the nails of my coffin to keep from going into the ground. I didn't find that edge in many other patients. Most people were much more placated by their doctors and their treatment. They didn't ask too many questions. I have always been a fairly aggressive person. I had this attitude—false as it was and still is—that nothing was too big, too tall, too far. If there is a task I'm not accomplishing, it is not because I cannot, it's because I don't want to. I was a cocky kid. Then cancer comes along and smacks me down to nothing. It swallowed me.

"With due urgency and extreme diligence, I began to attack this, all the time wanting to trust my doctors and nurses. Their idea of diligence did not match mine. They do this every day. It is their job. To them, I was not special unless I made myself special. I became the loudest dog in the pack, and I found it started to work.

"My care improves greatly if I have high spirits and keep an aggressive attitude. When my nurses stroll into my room, I am stern but happy. I project an attitude of 'I am the most important person that you are going to deal with tonight.' I put some humor into it, but I keep a strong presence about me so they are mentally aware of me. When my chart comes up in tumor board, my practitioners fight for me because I've made them remember me. I care and they know that.

> **"The only** finger I have wanted to point in my whole life is at the doctor who misdiagnosed my cancer."
>
> —Brian Lobel, 23

"Before going into an appointment or into the hospital, I always figured out within myself what I wanted to have happen. I had a decision tree. If my tumor is inoperable and this doctor will not operate, then I will ask for recommendations for another doctor. I won't use a doctor who is not interested in saving me. I don't want to come out of this asking, Who is a good funeral home director? I want to find out who is a good surgeon.

"There are two sides to a conversation with healthcare people. There is the personal side—they have to have some level of interaction with you, you are not an ATM—and the technical side. I'd be nice on the personal side until the technical side wasn't working my way, and then I'd get more and more stern and aggressive with the personal side. The volume of my voice increased as needed. I wouldn't yell or pound my fist. No desperation, but I didn't accept certain types of answers. I'd say, 'This is unacceptable,' and make them respond. I urge anyone in such a situation to use the word 'unacceptable.'

> "**They made** me sign a waiver in pre-op: I could die, bleed to death, have a hysterectomy. Doctors should discuss this with you beforehand instead of leaving you to sort it out with an orderly while your tears well up and the drugs start to kick in."
>
> —*Katie Smith, 37*

"My surgeon said, 'If we get in there and we can't get the whole tumor out, we are going to have to sew you up.' I said, 'No. Debulk it. You have to be able to get something out. Don't come out empty-handed.' Every time I have surgery, they need to remove a rib. It's like money on the collection plate. I wasn't going to tolerate this drastic alteration of my physiology without some attempt to save me. They say, 'Well, removing the tumor could spread disease.' I say, 'Who cares if it is going to kill me anyways?' A lot of people did not have that same attitude of, 'Do everything you can.' So many times, my care has tilted not on what the doctor thought but on what I thought. When the doctor says, 'I can't do this for you,' I just come back with two barrels and say, 'This is how it is.'

"I have coerced nurses and other staff into getting my films and putting my name on the top of the doctor's list. Here is how I do it. First example: 'If you can't find my paraffin blocks in your warehouse by tomorrow, my doctor is not going to want to operate on me, and I am going to die. So if you wait another few weeks to get this done, you won't be getting calls from me anymore because I'll be dead. But you will be getting calls from people who care that I am dead and are much more persistent than me, if you can imagine.' Another tactic is to find a way to flip the situation back on them. Second example: 'Ma'am, if I told you you were going to die, where would you stop to figure out how bad you wanted to live? Would you stop at this juncture right here, where I'm at, and you can't help me? Is that where you would stop? That is where I am. And I don't want to stop. And you are the person who has to help me.' You don't want people to pity you; instead, you want to empower them by putting them in a position where they can take pride in the feeling that they might have helped save someone today.

"I should never have lived this long. I don't know if it is my surgeries, my tenacity, or luck. Many people say, 'You are still alive because you have a purpose.' Everybody has their own belief system. I don't believe in that. People want to pour a lot of evangelism on this and give me big hugs and tell me how they are having prayer chains. But I see so many people lean on prayer for their strength instead of leaning on themselves; they don't grab the stinking reins of their illness and drive it into the ground, and they die. Prayer is never enough. It is not an answer. I feel it is a mechanism for coping.

"When I say grabbing the reins, I mean forget about fighting cancer; fight the doctors. Cancer does what it does. The cancer is evil and horrible and will kill you, but you have to respect the fact that it knows nothing other than trying to survive on its own. All cancer is trying to do is survive. It is a mutation. It isn't even an organism; it is part of you that thinks it is doing the right thing, so I cannot be mad at the cancer. I'm pissed off at the doctors for not getting my films in a timely manner, for giving me twice as much Ativan as I needed, for trying to put a cord needle instead of a Huber needle into a port. I'm ticked off the cancer shows up on an X-ray the size of a bottle cap, but they don't even call me until a year later when it takes up the size of a whole lung. I can't fix my body, but I can try to fix the problems with the people who could fix it for me."

"**I felt** like I had to fight for my right to be pain free. My nurses made me feel like a drug addict after my bone marrow biopsy. 'Nobody else needs pain killers,' they said, all condescending. Sorry, but I'm the boss of my own body."

—Dana Merk, 24

Greg's role as an aggressive advocate was familiar since I, too, had successfully challenged my doctors' protocols multiple times, changing the course of my care for the better. Nine months had passed in which the nodes in my neck either shrank or remained stable, and I was enjoying a quiet lull in my cancer care for the first time in four years. Since my original diagnosis, I had taken a nonstop hard-core approach to educating myself by reading copious amounts of medical literature from credible sources. I used reference guides that helped decipher complex terminology and crafted challenging clinical questions for my doctors that were far more advanced than the standard script of the 'five questions to ask your doctor when first diagnosed with cancer.' I found, however, that my greatest barrier was not in comprehending the science but in persuading my doctors to pay attention to me long enough to let me ask the questions.

As someone who told her fourth-grade Sunday school teacher to fuck off, I had never been daunted by authority. I used my years of improvisational performance training to play chameleon, adapting my approach from doctor to doctor to get them to listen to me and give me the answers I needed. Among these many tactics were pretending I was stupider than I am, dressing nicely for appointments, acting as if the reason I wanted my questions answered was not because I was a proactive cancer patient but because medicine seemed so cool and interesting, and restraining my emotions in front of doctors. Even though most of my charades were successful, I never felt as victorious as Greg sounded. I felt that in addition to losing my thyroid and thirty-one lymph nodes, I often lost a piece of my dignity by pretending to be someone other than myself, in order to get what I needed from people whose job it was simply to serve me. While speaking with Mary Ann a day earlier, I began to wonder whether part of the reason I was not taken seriously was because I'm a woman and young.

I succeed in not only challenging my doctors but also in scaling the fortress of hospital administration. Most healthcare administrators and office staff whom I encountered were there for a paycheck, and, unlike Greg, I found that extracting empathy from them was like squeezing water from a stone. The rare few who considered my medical care more important than office gossip were stymied either by their own incompetence or by institutional bureaucracy, which they, too, were unable to surmount. Despite these hurdles, I racked up hundreds of hours fighting for and winning the administrative battles on which my health hinged. My friends and family applauded my tenacity and know-how when navigating the system. Some suggested that I find nicer doctors or better-managed hospitals; however, the doctors and the administrators I was jousting with were from two National Cancer Institute Comprehensive Cancer Centers, which offer the best possible level of care in the country. Like Greg, I knew that the only way to improve the outcome of my disease and increase the quality of my care was to clearly and logically advocate for good health insurance, prudent medical decision making, and organized record-keeping

Greg continued to speak about his care needs, although this time it was directed toward his family. "I'm a very pragmatic patient, even with my friends and my family. When I lived at my parents' house after my lung surgery, I had a rule: no crying. I can handle my pain and suffering, but I cannot handle hearing my mom cry. Who can? Even if she just stubs her toe, I think, Oh, my poor mom is crying, somebody do something! I realized if I reacted like that when she was crying about me, I could spiral into a pity party for myself. Pity feeds on itself, and you can't get out of it. It is like depression. So I said, 'You and I can talk facts, we can talk survival, we can talk cold and blunt, but save your tears for your friends and my funeral. I can't hear it. Don't cry in the hospital. Don't cry here at the house or on the phone with your friends.' And she hasn't, not once ever. I've long since left their house, and I've asked her friends, 'Did she ever cry or worry about if I was going to make it?' They said, 'Oh, she did lots of that, but don't worry, Mr. Rules, it wasn't when you were around!'

"During the time I was at my parents' house, I came close to dying one night. It was evening time before dinner. I went upstairs to lie down because I just didn't feel good. The room became very, very still. I could hear the TV and my dad shifting in his chair and my mom cooking in the kitchen. There was a general amount of pain and malaise that I felt every day at that time, but that began to slip off and I began to feel myself cooling down. I was very still, but inside my head was an enormous amount of activity.

"**It sounds** cheesy and new agey, but I talked to the parts of my body that were in pain or going to be removed and I'd just cry. I absorb so much medical jargon and legal, financial, and administrative crap that I have to take time to regain control of my body."

—*Debbie Ng, 27*

"My mind might have set up this experience because it was copying what it had seen done in the movies, but I saw my life flash before my eyes. Scenes from my life, both good and bad, scrolled from left to right. Oh, there is that time at the lake; there is that person I hadn't seen in a long time. In some scenes I was first person and in others it was third person. And in my head, right beside me was a bucket that began to fill and I knew in a dreamish way that the bucket was full of regrets.

"Sometimes a feeling would pass that did not have pictures to go with it, like a clip of me and my high school girlfriend. Visually, it was blank, but it would cross my heart, almost like a reminder or an IOU of regret. The film slowed down, and the room started to cool. I had a bucket full of regret, but the bucket was just there, it wasn't the main thing. I think I was dying. I never experienced that before or since. I was so cold, but it was a great feeling. It was calming and relaxing, the most wonderful feeling I have ever had. It was incredible.

"I didn't even know if I would be able to get up, but I wanted to because I felt like if I didn't, I'd just pass away. I went downstairs and looked at my father. He checked my blood pressure and couldn't find any. He checked my pulse and couldn't find one. We jumped in the car, and he drove quickly to the ER. I ran in and was banging on the window of the triage. They checked me out. Nothing was wrong. Every single time I go to the emergency room, by the time I get there everything is fine, there is never a problem.

"I formulated a theory about two hours after I didn't die: all this stuff in your life, for years and years, boils down to about three minutes tops. It was a qualitative feeling, not quantitative. There was no metric with it. It wasn't how much do you have, how many friends do you have, or how many times you have done whatever. The question that arose when my whole life flashed before my eyes was, So how did you do? Did you do okay? And lumped into that is, Did you matter to other people? Did they matter to you? Were you good? That's what the secret to my life was. Those very basic questions. My life mattered. It was pretty good. But I could matter to more people in a much better way. I was so lucky to get that opportunity. I wish everybody could go through that and survive. It makes your life so much more . . . well, they all seem like cheap words to use for something so strong.

"One thing I decided to do—now this is going to come off wrong and could conjure some interesting images, but I decided to love as many people as I could. I want to matter where need be, not to go out and be evangelic about it or canvass as many peoples' lives as I can, but to just matter to people. I want to stop and notice people who matter to themselves, people who have dreams, who take themselves seriously and it is obvious.

"On the flip side, there are also people who just drain you, never get anywhere in life. They have a whole shelf of self-help books at home, and you just want them to stay home and read, instead of coming over to your house. It's been very hard, but over the past years I have also tried to wean these people away and get rid of them."

Like Greg, I had instituted what I coined the Drama-Reduction Program to rid myself of the drama queens and kings in my life. Cancer was a major crisis over which I often had no control, and I desperately want to squelch any ounce of additional calamity that I could. I dissolved relationships with high-maintenance friends and acquaintances. Although I felt guilty and selfish at first, the more I did it, the easier it became, and the results were phenomenal. As my physical and mental world spiraled out of control, I had downsized my social life into a group of even-keeled and low-maintenance friends who supported me.

Greg continued to talk about the other changes he enacted in his social life, as we hopped into his truck and headed to the airport. "After looking in that bucket, another big regret I have is playing around so much when I was younger and not rising to my potential and getting my MBA. When my friends were studying and working away, I was about fast cars, chasing skirts, top-shelf liquor, spending my money, and having a good time. I'm trying to make up for it now by teaching myself new things in engineering. I might not live for a whole long time, and I want to spend time doing some of the things that I really like to do. It has made me really selfish with my time, which has not worked out well for me in relationships. In a burgeoning relationship, you've gotta intertwine your lives. Gals who I'm dating are occupied with going to parties on a Saturday night, and things like that just feel trivial to me now, and I cannot make them impor-tant. I find I'd rather be home doing my laundry or going camping by myself on my boat in the middle of the lake, eating soup out of the can, reading *Jonathan Livingston Seagull*, and drinking a little rum.

"With cancer, I had experiences I didn't want to share with anyone. I wanted to set aside very small amounts of time each day to think about death. I said to myself, You can think about this at night, right before you go to bed. A little bit of that is healthy. You have to. You've got to let your emotions bleed a little bit. Sometimes it was frightening, and I'd worry. Sometimes it was tearful. It was always by myself.

"Since I have had my ribs out, I work on my sailboat with great care, I work hard at my career, I come home from work and read technical engineering books, I build HTML and surf the Web until 1 A.M. I do all of this because I will go to any length to keep from thinking about dying. Thinking about death frustrates me because there is no solution. I can't fix the problem. And it is always there. It is the dust on the floor at the end of the day. But the whole thing is that there *is* no problem. I think to myself, You're probably gonna die soon. Maybe a few years. What's up with that? I don't know what's up with that. I know what it is like to slip down that path, and it was great. I look forward to that. I couch death as a problem, but that is just it, there is nothing to solve so it cannot be a problem. It's a thing. What's the problem with dying? Well, nobody wants to. Well, that's not a problem; it's a statement. It is an inevitability, a singularity, a point you come to. Everything around me is normal, but inside me, this conversation continues and it never ends. It is a tumultuous mental affair that just wrecks my brain. It's not that it is morbid to think about death or it makes me go, 'Woe is me,' but it just doesn't serve me to do it. As a living person, death is the absence of that, so I cannot contemplate that. It is irrational.

"I have a dream that one of these days I'll take a year-long trip in my little boat to the South Pacific. Daydreaming about sailing is a great distraction, but eventually this little conversation takes place in my head so quick and fast, I'm talking to myself and having an argument with myself on the boat: I'm thirty-seven. That is pretty neat, Dawson. Didn't think I'd make it this far, and here I'm still kicking it. What about forty? Ever gonna make it? What if we don't make it? What good is this serving to think about death? I can't solve death, and I cannot avoid dying. I try to keep intense, stay on the edge, do all the fancy career stuff, do all my hobbies and interesting things to stay in the loop and keep from thinking about death. And that is why I don't think I'll ever go to the South Pacific, because what is going to happen when I'm in the middle of the ocean and it's not quite time to eat dinner yet, sails are set, and there is nothing to do. What are you going to do, buddy—think about dying? Maybe I'll keep the boat on the lake and buy a sports car instead."

As Greg approached the airport, I teased him, asking whether it made him nervous to drive in the "terminal departure" lane. Before we parted, he confessed that if he could go back in time and choose whether to get cancer, he would choose to have it. This was not the first time I had heard this response from a young cancer patient, but I was shocked to hear it from Greg, who actively tried harder than anyone else I'd met to advocate for his cure. I didn't tell him how sad and angry I felt every time I heard patients express that choosing cancer would have been the right choice. Had good things come from my own cancer? Yes, talking to Greg in his truck was one of many, but I believed that I was a pretty decent and self-aware person who did not need this horrific experience to make me appreciate the world around me or my role in it. If people needed pain through which to learn life lessons (and I debated whether that was even true), opportunities to open oneself up to suffering abound, and it saddened me that most people do not make themselves vulnerable in this way until they have no other choice.

On the plane ride home, I sat next to a woman who preached to me from the Bible, which distracted me from the anxious feeling of being stuffed in a sardine can. Shannon picked me up from the airport and drove me home to our apartment, which we had recently rented together. Our friends came over that evening to celebrate my thirty-third birthday. They crowded around the dinner table listening attentively to the details about who I met on my trip down south. It made me think that perhaps we as a culture are not afraid to talk about illness and death. Maybe we are just yearning for that window of opportunity to speak about them a little more openly and among friends.

RESOURCES

Working the System

Doctors make mistakes. Computers err. People are lazy. The health-care system is buckling. When I think about sparing my lungs from metastases, saving my vocal chords from unnecessary surgery, and getting the best treatment regimen possible, I approach the challenges of the system as if I'm on a personal vendetta. I crush the system like a superhero who has grown a hundred times my size. I sleep at night knowing I have done everything within my power to influence my outcomes. That is my definition of well-being.

Second Opinions

Most Americans will spend more time comparison-shopping for flat-screen TVs than searching for the best doctor possible. This is your life we are talking about, and cancer is not something to take lightly.

- Many insurance companies will pay for you to get a second opinion. Why? Because if you are misdiagnosed, it will cost them more money.
- When you get your second opinion, visit a doctor who is more specialized or has greater expertise than the first and who practices out of a cancer center with a higher volume of patients.
- Any good doctor expects that you will get a second opinion and will give you a referral to a doctor who is more specialized or more knowledgeable. If a doctor scoffs at your getting a second opinion, that is a huge warning sign.
- It is fair game to ask for a second opinion at any stage in your cancer—for example, a second opinion on your treatment regimen, a new drug, or if you have a recurrence.

Where to Find a Great Doctor

Take a three-pronged approach, and see whose name keeps popping up:

1. Get word-of-mouth referrals from doctors, nurses, and other patients who have your disease type.
2. Visit the home page of a top-notch hospital to see whether it specializes in your kind of cancer, and read bios of its doctors.

3. Scan journal articles on your disease to see whether an author's name appears frequently.

Beware of books and magazine articles that rank best doctors of the year or best doctors in your city. These sources are little more than popularity contests among doctors and should not serve as the sole source for finding a good doctor. Doctor referral and doctor scorecard Web sites run by for-profit companies are also unreliable sources.

When you receive any referral to a doctor, ask what criteria the referral is based on: Is the doctor on a referral list because he or she paid to be on the list? Is a doctor's name at the top of a list in a hospital's physical referral network simply because the computer rotates new names to the top of the list on a daily basis? If an acquaintance recommends a particular oncologist, do you know why he or she liked this doctor and are his or her standards the same ones you would use to evaluate who is the best doctor for you?

How to Rate a Doctor

- Ask your doctor: how many patients have you treated with my diagnosis and my stage? Ask surgeons: how often do you perform the kind of surgery I need and what is your success rate?

- Research online to determine how involved your doctor is in conducting clinical trials and cancer research, how often he or she has access to leading peers who are researching your kind of cancer, and whether he or she is certified.

- Visit the Web site www.pubmed.gov. Enter the name of the doctor in the search bar. This will show you any scientific research articles and papers he or she has published. Does this doctor have many (or any) publications listed? If so, how recent are they?

- Enter the doctor's name into a search engine to find an online biography. Is the doctor associated with a teaching institution?

Is he or she an active member in associations or medical societies that serve your disease? Does the doctor hold a noteworthy position within this organization that extends beyond simply being a dues-paying member? Does he or she present at conferences and how recently and regularly?

■ Don't forget to call 866-ASK-ABMS (866-275-2267) to find out whether the doctor is board certified.

How to Rate a Hospital

Most Americans will drive two hours to get a bargain at an outlet mall but will try to find the hospital closest to their house, rather than the best hospital they are able to get to. If there was ever a time that convenience should not be a top priority, this is it.

The gold standards are National Cancer Institute Comprehensive Care Centers (at www.cancer.gov search the "Cancer Centers List," or call 800-4-CANCER [800-422-6237]) and centers designated by the National Comprehensive Cancer Network (search at www.nccn.org for its member institutions, or call 888-909-NCCN [888-909-6226]). If you cannot be seen at a hospital on one of these lists, locate a university teaching hospital that is nearest you. If there are none, then larger hospitals (those with 200 to 500 beds) will give you better access to new technology, treatments, tumor boards, pathology labs, and diagnostic labs. Try to find a hospital that meets the guidelines of the American College of Surgeons' Commission on Cancer (at www.cancer.org, search "Find a treatment center," or call 800-ACS-2345 [800-227-2345]).

Communicating with Your Doctor

■ Doctors who are used to seeing patients three times our age may take for granted what we do or do not understand about health care, medical language, and how the system works. Ask for clarification if you need it.

- If an older adult accompanies you to appointments, some doctors may inadvertently exclude you from the conversation. Make sure they know that you are in charge.

- If your doctor truly sucks at communicating, type your questions out to hand to the doctor during your appointment. Sadly, some doctors relate better to objects than to people.

- If you are in a medical teaching hospital, capitalize on the fellows and the residents to be your conduits for communication with your doctor and to clarify any information that your doctor provides.

- Read "'Doctor, Can We Talk?' Tips for Communicating with Your Health Care Team," a fact sheet from CancerCare, www.cancercare.org, 800-813-HOPE (4673).

Time Savers

- Keep a cheat sheet in your wallet with all of your doctors' phone and fax numbers, your medical records number, and your pharmacy phone number.

- Have your doctor call in a prescription when you leave the office so that you don't have to wait at the pharmacy.

- Add caregivers' or friends' names to the HIPAA (Health Insurance Portability and Accountability Act) forms at your doctors' offices and hospitals. This will legally allow them to be able to talk to your doctors and other medical staff on your behalf.

- Contact your state Department of Motor Vehicles to see whether you qualify for a disabled-parking placard.

Know Who to Talk to

- Get to know your doctor's nurse and office staff. Be really nice to them whenever possible because they are key to making your administrative life flow smoothly.

- Most hospitals have a patient representative's office, a patient services office, or an ombudsman who can intervene on your behalf if you are not receiving timely or adequate service. Never hesitate to use them.
- If a patient representative or an ombudsman is not serving you satisfactorily, ask to speak to that person's supervisor and work your way up the chain of command; do not hesitate to call the office of the hospital's CEO because he or she is usually capable of making things happen swiftly.
- If you need to, file a complaint or at least threaten to file a complaint with your State Medical Board. Visit the Web site of the Federation of State Medical Boards, at www.fsmb.org, 817-868-4000; search the directory of State Medical Boards and link to or call your state board to file a complaint. You can also send a complaint, or threaten to send a complaint to the Joint Commission, a hospital accreditation organization. Call 800-994-6610 or email complaint@jointcomission.org.
- Stop at nothing to get your questions answered, the care you deserve, and the administrative support you need to make it all happen, but try not to do anything that would land you in jail.

Five Tips for Managing the Phone Call Maze

Use these tips when calling medical records departments, scheduling departments, insurance companies, and other bureaucracies.

1. Track all phone calls, noting date, time, name, location of the representative, and action taken.

2. Request that all of the information you have discussed (policy benefits, limitations, government regulations, or billing resolutions) be sent to you in writing.

3. Be aggressive, yet polite. People to whom you are polite will sometimes pull strings for you; people to whom you are rude rarely do.

4. Explain to phone representatives that you are young and living with cancer, which often yields sympathy that translates into favors and expedited requests.

5. Never hesitate to speak to a supervisor, a manager, or another person who is higher in the chain of command.

Best Desperate Measure

Read your hospital's philanthropy e-newsletter, and drop a donor's name in the lap of the CEO when you call to complain. After doing so, I had a team of techs spend the weekend scouring the back-up system for my ultrasounds.

11

Off the Map

When thirty-seven-year-old HollyAnna DeCoteau Pinkham called and told me about hiding her cancer diagnosis and treatment from her husband and parents, I knew immediately that I would purchase a plane ticket to Seattle and make a trek to the Yakama Reservation to meet her. Shannon and I had been dating for eleven months, and he had recently proposed to me. We decided that he would join me on this trip out West to celebrate our engagement and relieve some of the stress we accumulated during six weeks of investigating a spot on my lung (which was eventually found to be an error on the film, caused by the X-ray tech). Shannon would work in the hotel room during the days while I was with HollyAnna, and in the evenings we would indulge in all that the Yakima Valley had to offer us.

When I woke up at my best friend's house in Seattle, ready for our morning trip through the pristine, snow-packed Snoqualmie Pass, I still had no firm plans with HollyAnna. Each time I called to nail down a schedule, she would say, "Sure, call me in a week, a few days, a few hours, in another half hour." I began to wonder whether I was actually going to meet her. Midday, HollyAnna finally met us at our hotel in Yakima and was adamant that Shannon join us. Captive in her cramped car with tribal music blasting from the rickety stereo, we drove for four hours through the stark, rippling, gray foothills of her reservation. Our conversation was more like a guided tour of the land where she had been raised. We drove past the small wooden houses in which she had grown up, the Indian Health Services building, sweat lodges, churches, and dry winter farmland that in the summer produces hops and mint. When we passed the same post office five times, Shannon and I said nothing out loud but both realized we were driving in circles. HollyAnna seemed wired with untamed electricity. She spoke tangentially and at great length, and I knew I would need to scrub her rants of their chaos and disorder to make them readable by others.

"There is no word for 'cancer' in most Native American languages so I have begun to call it a shape shifter. In our language, a shape shifter is something that is evil and can change itself into any living form—a plant, an animal, a person. Its sole intent is bad, like the Catholic version of the devil. To me, this is the closest thing I can think of what cancer is. Cancer changes you, not necessarily for evil, but it is something evil that has come to you and is changing your life whether you want it or not.

"Most tribes believe that talking about illness can cause something bad to creep into the spirit, like you are opening the door for disease to enter your life. Cancer is like Dracula in the movies, who lingers outside a victim's bedroom but can't come in unless invited. With cancer, you know it is there, you know it exists, but it can't enter your little circle unless you invite it in. I'm not talking about it entering your physical body—your physical body can handle it. I'm talking about cancer entering your spirit, your will, the parts of you that there are no words to describe, that you can't see or hear or touch. That is what you are protecting from the cancer, and you protect yourself by not uttering the words.

"When I was twenty-five, I got cancer and I didn't tell anybody. Not my mother, husband, sister, or friends. I come from a traditional family so I dealt with it matter-of-factly by not acknowledging it. I told the doctors, 'Do what you've gotta do. Don't talk to me about it. I don't want to know.' I had melanoma, between stage II and III. I had surgery and took medication three times a day and successfully hid it all.

"I was married almost a year when I was diagnosed. My husband and I lived with his tribe on the Warm Springs Reservation in Oregon. We owned a house and had a seven-month-old son. It was my first real relationship. In my husband's eyes, we were newlyweds and everything was great. In my eyes, I thought everything that should be great was great, except for me.

"In order to hide the cancer, I had to be two different people, like how an actor must feel. My husband and I slept in the same bed, shared a home, and I never told him or anyone else. Sometimes I felt exhausted and my steroids blew me up like a balloon, but I had just had a kid so nobody thought different of it. My irregular job schedule as a paramedic and firefighter helped hide doctors' appointments. I threw away all of the prescription bottles and kept the pills in a little Altoids tin in my car. I kept the extra pills in sandwich bags in my coat pockets where nobody ever looked. Even though my son was only seven months old, I was constantly thinking, What if he finds my meds and accidentally ingests them?

"My specialist was in Bend, about fifty-some miles away. Many people who live rurally, farmers, low-income people, don't even have the gas money to go to get their treatments. I was lucky that I had a job and income and didn't have to worry about that. Living in a small community, people know each other's cars so I'd park in front of a restaurant, rather than in front of my doctor's office. My husband came to look for me at work one day, and I wasn't there. When I came home, he confronted me. I told him I was in Bend at an eye doctor's appointment. The day of my surgery I traded off an entire shift and did lots of little trades down the road, making it look like I was covering for someone who was sick. If anyone asked about the bandage, I'd say I had a mole removed on my arm.

"My doctors recommended that I tell my husband, but I told them no. I was flat-out resistant to telling anybody, though I did have one confidant; my baby was my little secret keeper. I took him to a lot of my appointments with me. I'd say to him, 'Don't tell anybody where we're going,' as if he could even talk. I told him stories about me growing up, about my life in case this thing became fatal. I thought even if he didn't remember my stories, he'd still have a sense of having heard my voice. I would tell him about the cancer, but I never actually said the word to him. It was so good having somebody to talk to and knowing that he wasn't going to tell anybody. I know he didn't understand a word of what I was saying, but it felt like he did.

"At that time, I didn't know anything about cancer, other than that's what my grandma died from. To me, it just meant dead or not dead. I wanted to be the not dead so I began exercising my tradition. I didn't tell people why I was doing it, but I started making teas, praying, fasting, going to the sweathouse, the medicine dance, the Sundance. People knew it was inappropriate to ask why I was doing all this, so they helped me, not knowing why they were doing it. When I was a child, my uncle told me, 'If you ever have what they call cancer, come get this plant at this time of year.' He taught me how to cure, treat, and prepare the plant. I look back and think, He said the word! I wonder if he knew something about my health that I didn't know.

"I did everything I could to remain strong and not think about why I was sick. Chopping wood and running were positive ways to deal with my frustrations and emotions because I'm not somebody who cries. I'm very good at maintaining neutral emotions. It takes a certain kind of person to work in public safety, where people are screaming, crying, or dying; their belongings are blowing up in flames; and everybody is running out of the burning building, and I am the one who is running in.

"In the back of the ambulance, people would give me their medical histories, and I started to wonder who else in my community has cancer and has never spoken about it. About five years after my diagnosis, I rode with a male patient who was an elder in the community. It was just the two of us in the back of the ambulance, and he told me that he had the illness. He told me, 'This is going to be my last trip. I will die at the hospital. I just want you to know that if I had told somebody earlier that I wasn't feeling well, I might be going to the hospital for a checkup instead.' That always stuck with me. I felt like he was telling me to speak up and make a difference. I've never forgotten that. I sang for him in the back of the ambulance and offered a prayer with tobacco. He died that night.

"He planted a seed in my head that these kinds of medical issues needed to be dealt with differently, but it took a while for the seed to grow. Cancer became something I didn't think about so much because my surgery was effective, my medications worked, and there were many other life-changing events that took place in my later twenties. My husband and I got divorced. I am sure that my lack of communication must have had an effect on our relationship. But we had many other problems, too. When I got divorced, I was in this limbo of, Who the hell am I and what am I going to do? Everybody thinks that cancer is the most changing thing in your life, but I think divorce taught me how to grow and change probably more than the cancer did. It made me be strong inside and encouraged me to speak up for myself. I got rid of my drinking buddies, and I started spending time with the elders. I moved back to the Yakama Nation in Washington, which is my native tribal land, and initiated a community-policing project. I wanted to be a leader.

"When I was thirty-five, I had a recurrence. My diagnosis was less severe than the first time. It was stage I. I needed laser surgery to remove the growth. The day before surgery, the nurse called to say, 'Don't eat anything after midnight,' only she didn't realize she was talking to my mom and not me. So I come home, and my mom asks, 'Surgery for what?' I'm like, crap, 'Mom, I have cancer again.' I'm hoping she can hear the 'again' part and think it went away once before so there is nothing to worry about, but she was completely freaked out."

HollyAnna hung a hard left and swung her car into the driveway of her family's house. She warned me and shannon not to mention cancer to her mom. She hopped out of the car and started into the house before we could ask any questions about our alibi. Her dad sat in the living room next to a huge Christmas tree, watching a Seminoles game on a large-screen TV. HollyAnna disappeared upstairs, while Shannon and I joined her mom, who was making beadwork at the dining room table. We gnawed on cured elk and stumbled over our words, dodging her questions about who we were and the purpose of our trip. HollyAnna eventually returned, diverting the conversation to a diatribe about curing with kosher salt.

The three of us piled back into HollyAnna's car. Shannon dozed in the back seat as we continued our circuitous route, with my tape recorder bumping on the dashboard. Her story was laden with holes that confused me. Later that night, as Shannon and I watched Yakima's Lighted Farm Implement Christmas Parade, I strategized about how to focus HollyAnna's scattered attention. The following day, I thwarted her lengthy itinerary of sightseeing and insisted that we meet in my room at the Red Lion Inn. Sitting at a tiny table strewn with beads, scissors, floss, and my recording equipment, she sewed and told meandering stories. I was not at all surprised when she told me that her native name Timal means "the sound of a woman working"; HollyAnna was a source of nonstop activity.

"After the surgery from my recurrence, I had to be still and rest my arm for ten days. I was completely bouncing off the walls. I was reading a stack of magazines and saw that the American Cancer Society was having a Western and Indian art auction to raise money. I wanted to donate one of the saddles I had made, but nobody from ACS would call me back. Fuck you, then, I thought. I'll have my own art auction. Lights went off in my head: this is how I'm going to make a difference for cancer in Indian country. So I just started calling around, getting connected, and learning that there are Indian cancer organizations. I began speaking about cancer with community members and even my elected officials at the state capital and in Washington, D.C. The seed that the dying elder had planted in my head in the back of the ambulance started growing wildly.

"I want to help people get screenings and detect their cancer earlier. I learned that Native American cancer patients often have a higher mortality rate than other cancer patients because it is discovered so late. It's not only because my culture doesn't speak about illness but also because of the unavailability of care. Most Natives get health care through Indian Health Service, which is run by the federal government as part of the treaty agreement to provide health and education to Native people. We have one tiny, single-story building on the reservation that serves ninety eight hundred people. They're understaffed and underpaid. Nobody wants to stand in line for eight hours to see a doctor. By the time you get in to see the doctor, you are still restrained by this very strong sense that females don't want to talk to males about their body and vice versa. There is a strong cultural barrier that inhibits screening. You just don't say to a stranger, 'I don't feel good,' or, 'There is something in my breast.'

This prohibits a lot of people from going to the doctors or even finding out about how to do a self-breast exam.

"It is hard to educate people in Indian country. You don't do it on the soapbox by telling other people what they need to do or by disseminating written information, plastering posters, or having little information booths. That doesn't work here, when tradition says you do not talk about your health point-blank. I knew I had to create a little hook to make people come to me. Make them ask me a question.

"I'm a jingle dress dancer. It is a specific dance that is done for healing, and you wear a dress that has rows of metal cones sewn onto it, as well as beadwork and other ornamentation. I sewed a beadwork patch onto my dress that said LAF. I'd wear my dress to pow-wows so that the other jingle dress dancers would come up and go, 'What is LAF? Those aren't your initials.' And I'd tell them about the Lance Armstrong Foundation, that I'm a two-time survivor, and about the importance of cancer screenings.

"That is how I started my education process. It worked way better than I thought it was going to. At my first pow-wow, I got over twenty questions. That was at least twenty times I got to say, 'I'm a cancer survivor.' Many of those people told me they had a spouse, a parent, a grandparent, a sibling, or a child who had cancer. That is when I realized that cancer in Indian country is a much bigger problem than I had thought.

"My family found out I was speaking about cancer in Indian country. I had a series of meetings that took place over weeks and months answering to grandmas, grandpas, aunties, and sisters. Some were opposed to me speaking publicly about cancer screenings, and a few were opposed to me going to the doctor in town. I said, 'What if I respect my culture and our traditional medicines and cooperatively take those, along with the medications of the white doctors? What if I put the best of both worlds together, and it can eliminate the cancer in me or in others in the community?' I have won over many of the family members, but it has not been an easy road.

"My heart is in the right place when I talk about cancer. Like when I am talking now in this conversation with you, Kairol. It is for good. So I pray that this doesn't bring evil in. I have the sweathouse, the medicine dance to ask for forgiveness for these actions. I have come so far in regard to talking about cancer, it blows me away. If I hadn't gone through it in silence the first time, I would now never be able to understand where the rest of my community members are coming from. I still get that voice in the back of my mind that says, If you say the word or if you talk about it, you are laying claim to it. I still never say it's mine. It is a thing, not mine. It is always 'the' cancer or 'the' disease.

"**George Burns** smoked cigars, drank alcohol, did crazy drugs, and died at a hundred and one. George Gershwin was one of the world's first popular vegans and died of brain cancer at thirty-nine. There is no rhyme or reason. The most important thing is to just own your lifestyle."

—*Matthew Zachary, 32*

"When I got cancer the first time, I was living in a bubble. I was in my early twenties, and I wasn't prepared to deal with it. I didn't know how to ask questions. I had a false sense of security and a blind faith in my doctors. I was in that in-between stage where you're not a youth, but you're not a full adult either. The second time around, I had grown up a lot more and was more secure in my identity. Now I know if I ignore a problem, it doesn't go away.

"I have changed greatly the second time around, but the mental aspects of living with disease are still very challenging. Not knowing how to slow down has been a lifelong weakness of mine. I've always been a multitasker, but it has become more extreme since the cancer diagnoses; I read a book, listen to the radio, and watch television simultaneously. I do these things to keep myself busy, to try to keep my mind off how the cancer is making me feel, mentally and spiritually, and to stop from wondering about the coulds, woulds, and shoulds.

"Sometimes when I'm starting to crash, I go to the mountains and watch the water. Water doesn't fight its way down the hill. It takes the path of least resistance. Still, there are rocks in the water, and that is how I look at cancer. It's a rock. I'll go around it, over it, under it if I can. I'm not going to fight it. Instead, I'll let it figure out how it is going to guide my path. You have to figure out how to work with the momentum cancer establishes in your life. Otherwise, you'll drive yourself nuts. So I have to go up to the mountains, and I remind myself that I'm like the water."

I could imagine HollyAnna at a medicine dance, blasting out e-mails about a community healthcare rally, or chasing after a criminal with a gun in her hand, but I could not imagine her lying quietly in the hills next to a stream. When I returned to Chicago and pored over the hours of our recorded conversations, these two sides of HollyAnna became clearer, as did the random bits of her story and the oddity of my time spent with her. I pieced together the reason we spent so much time in her car: it was the only private place to meet because she lived with her parents, there is no Starbucks on the reservation, and other public meeting places were tribal institutions in which it would be impossible to talk about the publicly forbidden subject of cancer. HollyAnna also spoke about her severe skin allergy to sunlight and mentioned fighting her insurance company to pay for a photosensitized windshield that made her car a UV refuge, where she could safely sit for hours on end.

HollyAnna had mentioned taking steroids, and as I began to research their side effects, it seemed plausible that they had contributed to her rushing energy. I called HollyAnna to ask her a long list of questions that would hopefully connect the dots of her scattered story. When we spoke, she had recently been taken off her medications. She was like a different person, with her attention focused and clear, her answers direct.

I wondered how many conversations I had recorded that were influenced by patients' medicated states of mind and how my impressions of them would differ had we met when either or both of us were healthy. I wondered what kind of lasting impressions I had made on people during the months when my high doses of thyroid medications affected my speech and energy level and deeply disori- ented my thinking. I so often defended against the idea that people living with cancer are different from those who have not experienced this disease. But maybe in some ways our personalities were very dif- ferent from others who had never had cancer and different even from our own personalities prior to cancer. Although insights and revelations may account for certain personality changes so often described by cancer patients, I suspected from my conversations with HollyAnna and from reflecting on my own illness that some of these shifts are instigated by the contents of a little orange bottle.

RESOURCES

Alternative Medicine

HollyAnna is an example of how difficult it can be to integrate two different forms of medicine into your cancer care routine and how much pressure others can put on you for the choices you make regarding your care.

When I was diagnosed, I was studying to be an acupressure therapist focusing on cancer, I had been vegan for seven years, and I trained as a dancer six days a week. People often ask me whether

I believe in alternative medicine. For me, medicine is not something to believe in (no one ever asks me whether I believe in my radiation treatment). Instead, it is something about which to ask, "Is it effective and will it improve my quality of life?"

Where to Start

Create a set of personal guidelines using these questions. Knowing your parameters for alternative care will save you time and energy.

1. What is my goal? (Reduce tumor size, ease the side effects of treatment, stress management?)
2. What can I afford and for how long can I afford it?
3. How much time per week can I dedicate to a regimen?
4. How far am I willing to travel?
5. Does this form of medicine need to mesh with my own concepts of spirituality or religion?
6. How much evidence do I require about the efficacy of the treatment?

Questions to Ask a Practitioner

- What are your credentials, and where did you receive them?
- How long have you been practicing, and what percentage of your clients have cancer?
- How and when will you determine whether the treatment is effective for me?
- What are the potential side effects of this treatment?
- Do you benefit economically from the treatment beyond your consultation fee? (Do you profit from the products you prescribe?)

■ If evidence-based alternative therapies are important to you, ask what studies are available, how were they conducted, were they reviewed or overseen by a reputable review board, how credible are the citations, and who are the other practitioners in the field researching this approach?

Alternative Medicine 101

National Center for Complementary and Alternative Medicine, www.nccam.nih.gov, 888-644-6226. This Web site provides tips for talking to your doctor about your alternative medicine choices; research and clinical trials on herbs, acupuncture, and macrobiotic and other diets; information on how to read dietary supplement labels; and much more.

Memorial Sloan Kettering Cancer Center: About Herbs, Botanicals, and Other Products. This site has extensive evidence-based information about herbs, botanicals, supplements, and more, including news and alerts about emerging research. Visit www.mskcc.org, and on the left-hand menu, click on "Cancer Information." When that page comes up, click on "Integrative Medicine" from the left-hand menu, and on the next page, click on the link called "About Herbs database."

Choices in Healing: Integrating the Best of Conventional and Complementary Approaches to Cancer by Michael Lerner (Cambridge, Mass.: MIT Press, 1996). Read this highly acclaimed book that teaches you how to think about and make choices regarding alternative medicine and cancer care.

Red Flags

Evaluate alternative medicine Web sites using the checklist on page 231.

Beware of anecdotes. They usually tell the stories of the few who have improved but do not mention those who diligently adhered to a regimen and died. Anecdotes are often based on the overly simplistic assumption that two events occurring at the same time have a cause-and-effect relationship. Other factors, however, such as allopathic (nonalternative) medicine, spontaneous remission, or environmental or lifestyle changes may be responsible for favorable outcomes.

Body and Mind

If you have limited time or money or are not interested in using alternative medicine, but still want to take a proactive approach to your health, these self-care practices can have a tremendous impact on curbing depression, reducing treatment side effects, and managing stress.

Exercise

Don't have time or money for the gym or classes? Walk with a friend, turn on the music and dance in your living room 'til you break a sweat, or use this excellent yoga book: *Healing Yoga for People Living with Cancer*, by Lisa Holtby (Lanham, Md.: Taylor Trade Publishing, 2004). Its yoga regimen was designed for people with all types of cancer and at any stage of the disease and includes safety guidelines for people who are in active treatment for cancer. Always talk to your doctor before engaging in these or any other exercises.

Sleep

Sleep is a free salve for the immune system. Carve out time to make sleep a priority.

Relaxation

Use CancerCare's downloadable fact sheet "Relaxation Techniques and Body-Mind Practices," which is available online at www.cancercare.org, or call 800-813-HOPE (4673).

Many cancer centers and organizations, such as Gilda's Club and the Wellness Center, offer free body-mind programs or may have lending libraries with visualization and relaxation tapes and books.

Nutrition

Cancer diets run the gamut from the straightlaced food pyramid to raw food diets. Do your homework to find a sustainable nutrition regimen that is right for you. Many cancer diets require making food that takes considerable time to prepare and may significantly add to your food bill. Consult your doctor any time you change your diet, and remember it is best to transition to a new diet slowly to allow time for your system to adjust.

Eating Organic

Eating organic foods is a great idea to reduce your pesticide intake, but buying organic groceries can take a serious toll on your wallet. Shop smartly.

Best to Buy Organic: Twelve Fruits and Veggies That Are High in Pesticides

- Apples
- Bell Peppers
- Celery
- Cherries
- Imported Grapes
- Nectarines
- Peaches
- Pears
- Potatoes
- Red Raspberries
- Spinach
- Strawberries

Best to Go Conventional: Twelve Fruits and Veggies That Are Lower in Pesticides

- Asparagus
- Avocados
- Bananas
- Broccoli
- Cauliflower
- Corn
- Kiwis
- Mangoes
- Onion
- Papayas
- Pineapples
- Sweet Peas

12

Naked in the Streets

My claustrophobic fear of flying, which I first noticed on my Alabama trip, continued throughout the following year. I wailed like a hysterical four-year-old, lying in a heap on the floors of airport terminals. Now my fear exceeded the limits of all shame. I was unable to board my flights, and I hyperventilated at the gates while the planes taxied and took off without me. My pathetic and irrational fear of small spaces swallowed my life, and I stopped traveling to meet cancer patients altogether. I succumbed to the landlocked Midwest, researching young adult cancer from my laptop, and tried to ignore my fear that this book would abruptly end a few chapters shy of completion.

My friends blamed wedding nerves as the culprit and suggested that my claustrophobia would pass after the big day. Wedding planning was a stress that paled in comparison to cancer, and Shannon and I were quite confident about our marriage. After a fifteen-year dating career, you know when you've got something good. Our wedding was a weekend filled with close friends and family, square dancing and Southern food, tapas and a swing band. The ceremony left the rabbi asking for a transcript, and the hora was fit for the *Guinness Book of World Records*. The wedding was not, however, an end to my claustrophobia.

I chalked up my claustrophobia to a clichéd textbook case of post-traumatic stress disorder caused by six years of my head being clamped into hockey mask–like cages and strapped in neck cradles, shoved into MRI machines, and sent through the doughnut holes of PET and CT scanners. After ten sessions of cognitive counseling for claustrophobia, the therapist and I agreed that it wasn't working. Anxiety was bleeding into my daily life, and she suggested antianxiety medication, which I flat-out refused. A second therapist pinpointed my anxiety as a side effect of my thyroid medication. Despite my repeated explanations that high levels of thyroid hormone slowed my cancer growth, she badgered me about lowering my dosage as a treatment for anxiety. I chose claustrophobia over fueling my cancer growth and never returned to her office.

I was furious that my doctors had failed to warn me about the side effects of my thyroid medication, yet I could have easily researched these side effects online and chose not to. I had rationalized, "Why give credence to side effects that are unavoidable and come with the potentially huge payoff of slowing cancer growth?' But my anxiety felt like a thick, smothering pillow pressed hard to my face that I could no longer ignore. I wished I could be like Tracy and embrace the mental complexities that accompanied my cancer, but when it came to depression or anxiety, I was more like Archie Bunker, with a stubborn, pull-yourself-up-by-the-bootstraps attitude.

I had three options: lower my thyroid meds, take antianxiety meds, or explore alternative treatments such as rapid eye movement desensitization. I convinced myself to take antianxiety medication by creating a justification that medication (rather than my own brain chemistry) caused the anxiety in the first place; therefore, medication should be used to counteract it. My general practitioner prescribed an effective pill, and within a month I was one-tenth of the freak I had become. This was very good timing because she also ran a blood test on my tumor marker and discovered that my cancer was back in full force.

When my friends said, "At least, cancer must be easier the second time around because now you know what to expect," they could not have been more wrong. Torturous memories of my first diagnosis were etched in my brain and actually worsened the anticipation of more surgery and treatment. Yes, I had learned lessons from my first cancer experience and from every patient in this book, but no state of mind or body of thought could eradicate the physical suffering that is cancer's baseline, and I knew that plenty lay ahead.

What did, however, make cancer easier this time was Shannon. Plunging into months of circular phone calling to nurses, doctors, and medical records departments, Shannon assumed the administrative burden of my cancer. He became a master researcher on new approaches to treatment and attended every appointment, grilling my doctors for new information. He was available to comfort me 24/7, and on days when I collapsed with exhaustion and fear, he walked our dog Moses, made spaghetti dinners, did the laundry, and ran our errands. He managed this routine while working a full-time job that offered top-notch health insurance, which paid for our travel, lodging, and care at the best cancer centers in the country.

I had became one of those married cancer bitches with a loving husband, whom I had been jealous of for so many years. My envy was completely justified; this was a status to desire badly and be grateful for when you had it. I had read that some patients experience guilt over putting their spouses through the suffering of their cancer. Guilt in this situation seemed like a waste of good luck, so instead I felt appreciation and knew that were the tables turned, I'd do the same for him. It sucked to have cancer three months after our wedding, but neither Shannon nor I was naive enough to think that happiness is untouchable. We were tired, pissed off, and sad, but we knew that this was life and we would figure it out together.

Shannon and I, with the help of a forward-thinking oncologist, devised a six-month alternative medicine regimen to shrink my slow-growing tumors. I gagged on dehydrated greens, downed shooters of frozen shark extract, took off-label diabetes medication, received acupuncture, and ate a high-fiber vegan organic diet that scraped my intestines, caused internal bleeding and extreme lethargy, and dropped me to my ninth-grade weight. I tortured myself on a daily basis by reminding myself how lucky I was to have a slow-growing form of cancer and wondering whether I was doing enough to try to stop it.

> **"Anyone who** deals with cancer as a chronic disease knows that it is a lot more complicated than just fighting one battle and winning."
>
> —*Rick Gribenas, 28*

At the end of six tiring months, I learned that my tumors were still growing and I would need immediate surgery in San Francisco. The same day that I received this news, Moses was diagnosed with cancer, too. The prospect of my dog dying from cancer while I was under the knife halfway across the country dislodged from my gut an exorcistlike force that had been swelling for six months. I threw myself on the floor in a shrieking tantrum. Twenty minutes later, I regained control and went on autopilot for the next six weeks.

I became extremely matter of fact. I obtained information, made decisions, wrote to-do lists for my parents, and flew with them and Shannon to San Francisco for my surgery. I arranged to meet with nurses, the anesthesiologist, and a chaplain. I told few friends I was in town and e-mailed and talked on the phone to almost no one for a month during my recovery. I swallowed my physical pain and popped a pill at the slightest twinge of anxiety. Although it was no piece of cake, this surgery was shorter with a quicker recovery than my first.

I knew that if I stopped working, I'd fall into the hole that had consumed me for two years during my original diagnosis and treatment, when purpose was absent and motivation intangible. I had begun a choreographic residency in Chicago and returned to the studio just a few weeks after my surgery. While I slowly regained mobility, I choreographed from a chair, imagining movement in the space. I hid my

> "**Cancer is** viewed as a war, but I've replaced that with a work analogy: illness is my second job. I go to the hospital, do my work, and come home."
>
> —*Rick Gribenas, 28*

cancer from everyone in the dance community in order to dodge pity, disbelief, comments about how heroic I was for making myself work during such a hard time, or sentiments about how healing the arts are in the face of illness. I was simply throwing myself into my work because I knew it would keep at bay the insanity that often comes from thinking too much about my cancer.

Writing this book was at times a haven from, and at other times a magnification of, everything I wanted to forget. I wrote furiously for days in a row, followed by a week or two when thinking about my or anyone else's cancer felt like sheer hell. During those stretches of time, I retreated to the couch with Moses (who was also recovering from cancer surgery) and numbed my mind with back-to-back *Law and*

Order episodes and *Project Runway* marathons. This was the first time in my adult life that I owned both a TV and a couch. Those empty TV days were also the first time as an adult that I had allowed myself to be completely unproductive without worrying about the consequences. In the end, I was much more productive than I would have been if I had forced myself to work when all I wanted to do was crawl into a hole.

I needed to talk with another young adult patient who worked in the cancer field to see how he handled this dual relationship. I arranged a conversation with thirty-two-year-old Matthew Zachary, a twelve-year brain cancer survivor who was the executive director of the budding nonprofit I'm Too Young for This (a.k.a. i2y). I had met Matthew over the phone a few months prior to my recurrence when I became the senior oncospondent for *The Stupid Cancer Show*, an interactive talk-radio show produced by i2y. Matthew had recently achieved a long list of accomplishments, ranging from i2y being ranked in *Time* magazine's top fifty Web sites of the year, to playing himself as a character on the Lifetime network TV docudrama *Side Order of Life*. What I found most compelling about him was not his growing glam, but his willingness to voice controversial perspectives on cancer; he was not just another good old boy in the cancer network.

I flew to New York claustrophobia-free, thanks to a stash of Xanax prescribed by my general practitioner. For our first face-to-face meeting, I visited Matthew at Mirrorball, an ad agency in Chelsea that provided him with pro-bono office space. The elevator doors parted on a post-punk, vintage loft space with peeling paint. As Matthew and I settled down in a cozy corner office, which sported skateboards on the walls and was piled high with art books, I felt like Dorothy meeting the man behind the curtain.

"I say I'm living beyond cancer. It left my body but didn't leave my life, and just because I'm disease free doesn't mean I'm cured of the experience. I try to position cancer as a life sentence, rather than a death sentence. Unless you are very lucky and have a quick in-and-out experience, you might be like me, dealing with post-traumatic stress and long-term physical side effects.

"There are so many inequities and injustices of the whole cancer situation. The institutionalized process leaves you naked in the street. When you are done, there is no one to catch you, pick you up, or cradle you through a continuum of care. After treatment, I was given no career counseling, social work, or peer support. When my friends and I graduated college, they all went to grad school, leaving me all alone to recover from aggressive full-body radiation. Treatments twelve years ago were horrible. I lost a hundred and ten pounds in three months, I was throwing up ten times a day, crippling headaches, pain, a wrecked esophagus, erectile dysfunction, infertility, hypothyroid, my skin was burned. I had temporary pre-glaucoma. I was manic. I had wanted to go to UCLA grad school to become a composer for film and TV scores, but after treatment I didn't want to write music anymore. I was done with the hope that I could reclaim what was lost.

"I just wanted to find work to get out of my parents' house on Staten Island. My bedroom there, the smell of the house, everything reminded me of treatment. I was so afraid to go into Manhattan and get a job because my immune system was really fragile, but when you are twenty-two, you just want to do your shit and get on with life so I bit the bullet. I got a job doing tech support for a pharmaceutical ad agency. I was so socially displaced. I was around strangers, which was both comforting and isolating at the same time. I was sick a lot, and it was really hard to go in to my boss and tell him about my cancer. I just wanted to be a good employee.

"**They send** around a memo at work when someone is sick so you can send them a card. I didn't want that done for me, but my boss felt it would make her look bad if she didn't. So she did."

—*Jill Woods, 38*

"After a year and a half, I moved on to my next job, which was more in the creative-marketing side of things. I started to make new friends and get a grip on my cancer. I also started to see a great therapist, who was a tremendous help. I wrote some songs about my cancer experiences and had a show at a club. I was so nervous, but after the show there was not a dry eye in the house. I printed a bunch of CDs and gave them away to friends and patients at hospitals. Drug company reps saw my CD at the hospital and asked me to do some spokesperson work. I had to stop and really ask myself if I wanted to go back into the cancer world. It was very Al Pacino–like; they pulled me back in.

"All of the drug companies started to ask me to speak at dozens of events. I didn't know what I was doing, I wasn't media trained. The PR folks would introduce me: 'Concert pianist Matthew Zachary was diagnosed with brain cancer at age twenty-one after losing use of his left hand. He is here to play the music he wrote when he was told he'd be dead.' Come on, you can't beat that. It became very motivational, very inspirational. I quit my job and began computer and marketing consulting so I could travel to these cancer speaking events. It brought me back into cancer from a different perspective 'cause now people were looking to me for help.

"I was discovering advocacy, how to work on behalf of other people who can't do it themselves. Slowly, over the course of years, I learned and listened. I met Doug Ulman from the Ulman Cancer Fund for Young Adults, Heidi Adams from Planet Cancer, and people at the National Cancer Institute. I became the go-to guy because I built an enviable Rolodex of cancer contacts. I taught myself about policies and what was really going on in the cancer world. I read *From Cancer Patient to Cancer Survivor: Lost in Transition*, a report about how screwed we are because the entire public health continuum is set up for the acute side of cancer and so ill-equipped to deal with it from a long-term perspective. I read *Closing the Gap*, about how young adult survival rates have made no progress in the last thirty years and are largely the same as when Elvis died. That is what really tipped me off that age matters in cancer. I developed a very irreverent attitude; if you are fifty, screw you, I've gotta be about young adults because no one else is.

"i2y started as an over-gloried Craigslist: Matt's favorite cancer sites for people under forty. Boom, it was an instant hit. It was cart before the horse. I didn't have a business plan for i2y; I just knew it would work because it was filling a need. It is a really simple Web site that made a really big difference in the cancer world by letting doctors, nurses, and patient navigators know that there are resources out there for their twenty-two-year-old patients. Before i2y, they could only tell patients to do a Google search; now they have a credible brand that connects young adults to all the resources they need.

"I started something really big unintentionally, but the lesson is that I did it smartly. I took my time, I listened, I identified gaps. It wasn't about raising money; it was about raising awareness and unifying a community that didn't know it existed. It is so easy to say I want to help, but most people help for the wrong reasons; they do it out of their own emotional need and duress, with no real thought into planning or analyzing what is most helpful, useful, and what actually needs to be done. If you want to help cancer, do not start a race and do not start a nonprofit organization. Starting and managing a nonprofit is an arduous, expensive, and long process. Everyone expects people to come out of

"**Maybe the** cure needs to suffer a bit so we can address the cause. There was so much rage over three thousand people dying on September 11, which was a great tragedy, don't get me wrong. But seventy thousand young people a year get diagnosed with cancer. Where's the outcry? Where's the 'We are gonna get whatever's doing this'?"

—*Geoff Luttrell, 35*

the woodwork and donate simply because you have nonprofit status. Oh, the money will flow! A lot of the work that is intended to help the cancer community ends up being duplicative, steals from the limited pool of resources, and raises funds that don't have an actual impact. People are stupid, they don't think, they act on impulse and without accountability. People don't think about these issues logistically because they get very primal and very territorial about, 'Cancer happened to me, and only I can fix it.'

"Here are three hypothetical examples of what to do instead of starting your own organization: One, if your mission is to help patients feel good about themselves through yoga, you don't need to be a nonprofit organization to do this. Just go to a yoga studio and ask them to work with you to offer discounts or free classes to cancer patients. Two, if you want to raise money and start a fund for your doctor who is doing his little research on X disease, don't do that. Instead, give that money to an existing organization with the most accredited, evidence-based research and longitudinal results that impact X disease. Three, maybe there is a group that funds better beds in the hospital, but you want to fund better bathrooms in the hospital. Get over yourself. Don't start another organization; instead, work with the existing hospital fund-raising department and tell them you want a fund for better bathrooms.

"My goal with i2y is not to just start yet one more nonprofit organization. My goal is to look at the root of the problem and create change. I lay awake at 3 A.M. wondering how we are going to make the next thirty years of cancer different for young adults. One reason that our survival rates have not improved is because we get diagnosed at stage III or IV instead of stage I or II. Signature gala events and walk-a-thons aren't going to change this predicament. Branding a national young adult cancer movement and developing wide-scale marketing to a targeted audience will make a real change in young adult cancer. How? Through smart social media campaigns we can make aware to both young adults and doctors that when a twenty-two-year-old presents symptoms of cancer, yeah, this might be cancer. What's happening now is that the young adult and the doctor are thinking, This has to be everything but cancer because she is so young, and then she isn't diagnosed until stage III. This kind of change isn't about scientific research or programming; it is about mass communication. While it is incredibly useful to have a nonprofit organization out there raising a hundred thousand dollars to give people rides to treatment, and I'm very glad that exists, I am more interested in working as a social entrepreneur to create a new movement that results in lasting social change in how the public relates to and engages with this disease in young adults.

"My attitude about cancer and the work that I do in this field is not an accident; it is the result of a twelve-year project. I was not like this much of that time. I didn't own my disease, I didn't have the confidence or articulation to talk about it. Owning my disease means I'm accountable for my history, I'm not ashamed of it, I'm responsible for the actions I took to get where I am at today. Twelve years ago, they told me I had a 50 percent chance of living for five years without chemo, and with chemo it would get me up to 55 percent. My doctors strongly advised the chemo, and I was like, 'Go fuck yourselves, no way.' Tell a seventy-five-year-old they have an extra 5 percent chance of living five years, but I'm twenty-one! So I didn't do it. I'm confident in those actions and decisions and have pride in what I am today. These are my experiences and no one else's, and I am

"**I tried** to escape the reality of my diagnosis with a shopping spree but the pink products were constant reminders. What I used to think was innocuous marketing now seems a manipulative device for preying on people's emotions. I'm glad money is being raised but companies are profiting off our illness and it is repugnant."

—*Jill Woods, 38*

not a victim. But this attitude probably didn't develop until six or seven years after my diagnosis. It just took time. Things just take time.

"The medical side of cancer is still a part of my life every single hour of every single day. I'm on military patrol with myself. I take my meds, see my fourteen doctors, and do what needs to be done. Some people use alternative medicine as their proactive care. My job is my proactive care. I'm living my passion and my dreams. I've turned myself into a career. And no, I never have days when I'm sick of thinking about cancer."

After three hours of rapid-fire conversation with Matthew, I headed to the New York Public Library to squirrel away and write. On my subway ride, I thought back to when I first started writing this book. I had asked Barbara Brenner, the executive director of Breast Cancer Action, for an important question she wanted me to pose to cancer patients. "What is it really going to take to cure cancer?" was the question she gave. Matthew had the answer. What it would take to cure cancer was more people who knew that an arsenal of compassion, money, heartfelt effort, and deep desire didn't mean much if you are not willing to put smarts and strategy above your own personal agenda.

RESOURCES

Making a Difference

Biking or walking for cancer research can be worthwhile, but the single most important action you can take to improve the survival rate of young adult cancer patients is to work toward increasing our access to quality, affordable health insurance.

While children and older adults have enjoyed a steady increase in survival rates since the early 1970s, the overall survival rate for young adults has not budged. The fact that many of us lack adequate health insurance is a key reason why we are diagnosed at more advanced stages that can carry a worse prognosis.

Young adults are the largest group of uninsured adults in the United States. According to the Commonwealth Fund, 13.7 million Americans between the ages of nineteen and twenty-nine do not have health insurance. (That figure is greater than the populations of New York City and Los Angeles combined!) The American Cancer Society's CEO John R. Seffrin declared, "If we don't fix the health care system, that lack of access will be a bigger cancer killer than tobacco. The ultimate control of cancer is as much a public policy issue as it is a medical and scientific issue."

Our access to quality, affordable health care is dependent on the government's passing laws to stop the health insurance companies from placing limitations on our care. For example, laws in various states now require insurance companies to allow children to remain on their parents' insurance until age twenty-five or in some cases thirty.

Use Your Voice

Connect with state or local organizations that are working to pass laws to expand health insurance coverage for young adults. You can offer these organizations what most other volunteers cannot: your compelling personal story of navigating the healthcare system as a young adult with cancer. These organizations will educate you about the specific bills they are trying to pass and will train you on the targeted actions you can take, such as making phone calls, writing letters, or meeting in person with your elected officials to tell your story and to discuss why you think the bill must be enacted.

> Until Washington D.C. steps up to the plate to provide health care to all Americans, the biggest changes in access to healthcare will continue to come from legislation at the state level. Get involved

with a healthcare action organization in your state. Visit www
.uhcan.org and select "state connections." Click on your state for
a list of local organizations where you can volunteer.

Visit Children's Cause for Cancer Advocacy (CCCA) at www
.childrenscause.org and click on "Take Action." CCCA's efforts
increase care not only for children but for twenty- and thirtysomething patients as well.

The American Cancer Society Cancer Action Network (ACS
CAN) is the non-profit, non-partisan partner advocacy organization of the American Cancer Society. As one of its many advocacy
efforts, ACS CAN has championed Michelle's Law, a bill to ensure
that college students cannot be dropped by their parents' insurance providers if they need to take a medical leave from school for
up to twelve months. Visit www.acscan.org, select "Campaigns"
and click on "Access to Care Campaign." Also, join ACS CAN's
Mobile Action Network to receive campaign and event updates,
as well as action items on your phone. Send a text message with
the words "Fight Back" to 73585.

Checklist for Twenty- and Thirtysomethings Call to Action

Use this checklist to make sure that the organization or legislative proj-
ects for which you volunteer will help young adults gain access to care.

- Does the legislation you are working on pertain to Medicare? If
  so, it will only serve those who are sixty-five and older.
- Will the legislation make health care affordable for people with
  low or moderate incomes? The average income for twenty-five
  to thirty-four year olds is approximately $35,500 a year.
- Does the proposal expand access to health insurance and
  increase its affordability?

- Has the organization you are working with promoted any legislation that pertains specifically to young adults age eighteen to forty?

- If you are working on legislation to make cancer screenings more available, do the medical screenings apply to patients under forty?

Use Your Vote

If you are not registered to vote, do so at the Web site www.rockthevote .org. Going to the polls to vote, however, does not mean jack for the fate of young adult cancer if you vote for a candidate who will allow insurance companies to deny care to young adults with preexisting conditions.

Don't just vote; vote smart. Visit the Web site www.votesmart .org and click on "Candidates." Follow the prompts to read about the candidates in your region and their positions on expanding health care. Whose side are they really on: yours or the insurance company's?

Use Your Mind

If you have ever complained about rising healthcare costs, it is your duty to understand how the healthcare system works and what you can do to change it. You do not have to be a policy expert to understand healthcare issues. Start by reading the reports below; the more you read the more empowered you will become as you begin to better understand health insurance language and issues.

- "Rite of Passage: Why Young Adults Become Uninsured and How New Policies Can Help," published by the Commonwealth Fund. Visit www.commonwealthfund.org and enter "rite of passage" in the search box.

■ "Health Insurance Coverage of Young Adults: Issues and Broader Considerations," published by the Urban Institute. Visit www.urban.org and enter "young adult insurance" in the search box.

Best Use of Your Time

Signing petitions and telling your healthcare story on action blogs are good fun, but aids on Capitol Hill advise that these forms of action are not effective in persuading lawmakers. The most effective action you can take is to meet in person with your elected officials. The second most effective action is letter writing followed up with a phone call.

13

Fluke

I could not organize in my mind or communicate to others the complexity of my health status. I wavered between saying "I have cancer" and "I had cancer." When a new doctor in Chicago decided that I could forgo my surgeon's recommendation for radiation, I did little to dissuade my family when their ecstatic e-mails concluded that I was cured. The doctor and I agreed that treatment had done little to successfully eradicate my cancer in the past, and the risks now outweighed the benefits. Friends, acquaintances, and family members asked, "Are you in remission?" "Have you completed treatment?" "Are you cancer free?" I gave pat responses because the truth required elaborate and technical answers that were beyond the reach of their simplistic, well-meaning, and somewhat clichéd concepts of cancer and remission.

Two tumors were found nestled on my jugular vein just a few months later. "You have more cancer" sounded par for the course to my ears, but the rest of me never got used to receiving the bad news. Was I supposed to cancel my dinner plans, call my friends, or send a group e-mail? I had no idea how to act or feel this time around, when my cancer was no longer fresh and startling news but rather tedious and redundant. Sitting on a radiator on the bridge that connected the hospital and the parking garage, I bawled on the phone to my mom. With each diagnosis, she had shed more of her overwhelming anxiety and became resolute that we had figured out a way to deal with it in the past and we would again.

With radiation being a non-option, my doctor deferred to my surgeon. Naturally, he wanted to operate, despite concerns that further surgery would shift my veins, arteries, and other neck structures and coat them with scar tissue, which would make imaging a challenge to decipher and successive surgeries a nightmare to perform. After seven years of attempting to cure this problem with surgery and treatment, I needed a doctor who would not only provide different answers but would see a different problem.

Matthew Zachary connected me to a doctor at Memorial Sloan Kettering, who was covered again by Shannon's uber-insurance. The doctor concluded that I would always have thyroid cancer. There was no cure for me. My survival rate was great, but I should always expect to live with cancer in me. Radiation was not an option, and we would also forgo surgery until the size of the tumors outweighed the risk of surgery. The chance of metastases to my lungs and bones was present but low.

It was simultaneously painful and deeply relieving to hear the sucky truth after seven years. An image lodged in my mind that hit me five years earlier when I received bad test results: on a mid-seventies episode of *Sesame Street*, Grover, dressed as a waiter, bursts through the swinging kitchen doors into the front of the house and slams down a ginormous hamburger two times the size of the table. Receiving news that I could not swallow or even take a bite of was like having that *Sesame Street* hamburger thrust on my plate. I was not in denial, but it would take me a good long while to gnaw away at and digest the truth.

The stress and the exhaustion of repeatedly traveling to Sloan Kettering wore me down. Although I would continue indefinitely having one-on-one conversations with random young adult cancer patients, I had an editor who needed my final manuscript in a month and I wanted to meet with a patient for whom fertility issues was at the core of their cancer experience. For privacy reasons, I had thus far been strict about patients finding me, but I needed to change the rules to accommodate the insanity of my last few weeks. I cold-called Dana Merk, who had been diagnosed four years previously at age twenty-one with a form of acute myelogenous leukemia that is most often found in sixty-five-year-olds.

> **"Me and mother** have become not just mother-daughter but best friends. It seems like our brains are connected because we think and say things at the same time. Our closeness is probably because of my cancer but also because I'm getting older."
>
> *-Krista Hale, 39*

She lived in the Chicago suburbs, and when I explained the status of my life, she volunteered to meet me at my apartment. Sitting on my couch in my living room was an odd and somewhat vulnerable reversal. Dana was an open book, and for four hours we talked nonstop, laughing and busting out the Kleenex.

"When I talk about my cancer, I don't say this is what I went through, I say this is what we went through. My mom was with me every single hour of every single day. She was my everything, my buddy, my best friend, my wingman, my rock. We slept in the same room together for a year. My mom wiped her twenty-one-year-old daughter's ass for a year 'cause I couldn't reach it with my central line. That is love. The night I was diagnosed, I was consoling her, 'Mom, I'm going to be fine.' But there was no consoling her because this is every mother's worst nightmare.

"My mother turned into a mama lion who had to protect her young. We were in the hospital for six weeks, and she kept her own log and wrote down everything that entered my body and what my reactions were because mistakes happen all of the time. My mom put a big sign on my door: Do NOT wake my daughter up at 5 A.M. to weigh her—she is sick! They paid attention to my mom because she is a little Italian bulldog, and she'd kick their ass if they didn't. She was tough, but she also knew how to make me laugh. I was in the hospital, nauseous and shitting my brains out, and you hear over the loudspeaker, 'Code red, code blue.' My mom is putting her gloves on, saying, 'We've got a code brown over here!'

"When people ask me now how I managed to get through that time, I always play it down because I don't want pity. 'Oh, it wasn't that bad,' I say. If my mom hears that, she's like, 'Were you in that room? How many times did you almost lose your life?' I was going through it, but she had to witness it, and I think that was a lot harder. There are no mirrors in the ICU; I couldn't see what I was going through. She sat and watched the monitors without blinking. Her pain was just as deep as mine, and I think she went through a lot more than I did.

"She tried to be strong for me and in front of me. Once or twice, when we were back home, I found her upstairs on her knees praying, sobbing, bargaining. It was the worst thing ever. She says, 'You will not understand what I'm going through until you are a mom,' and I agree. Even now, I cannot imagine how hard it must be for the caregiver to be so absolutely helpless. She would have switched places with me in an instant if she could.

"I cannot wait to be a mom so I can feel that scary love that moms feel. I want to be able to understand what she went through. I have wanted to have kids as far back as I can remember. My mom has always said I give off a scent, a pheromone that makes babies clamor to me. I think that being pregnant, being in labor, and giving birth has to be one of the coolest things ever. I was in Macy's the other day trying on a cute smocky dress, and since the fitting room was next to the maternity department, there was a tummy pillow form hanging on the wall. I tried it on under the dress and paraded in the mirrors, checking myself out, pretending I'm pregnant. It is demented and obsessive, but my life and being a mom are interchangeable.

"My mom and I both knew to ask the doctors about fertility when I was diagnosed, but it fell on deaf ears. We had to start chemo, and they said, 'Isn't your life more important than your fertility?' I couldn't be a mom if I was dead so I started induction chemo, which risked ovarian failure. They didn't care so much about chemo affecting my ovaries because I was in a clinical trial that had an autologous stem cell transplant scheduled five months down the road, and that was the real deal that would have made me permanently infertile.

"After the induction chemo, I sought out a fertility specialist on my own. My mom

> "**I needed** to meet a man, get married, and start a lengthy surrogacy or adoption process. I had a ticking clock even though it wasn't truly biological."
> —Katie Smith, 37

> "**I woke up** in the recovery room and my doctor informed me I had cancer and an unexpected complete hysterectomy. Her stomach was at my eye level and she was six months pregnant. It was like adding insult to injury."
> —Katie Smith, 37

> **"At the sperm bank** I had a private room with a sexy leather couch that I sat on until I realized how many other people must have masturbated on it. There were no videos, only a soft-core poster and a bunch of *Playboys*. I was kind of disappointed."
>
> —*Brian Lobel, 23*

and my boyfriend came to the appointments with me. None of it was covered by insurance, which sounds like it should have been a big deal, but at that time money seemed small compared to the other life-threatening issues we were facing. Debt was something we could deal with later. I couldn't enroll for the spring semester when I was in the hospital so my mom's insurance plan dropped me because I was twenty-one and not a student. We had to take out COBRA, which was a shit ton of money, and my mom was on an unpaid leave of absence from her job as a court reporter so she could take care of me. People emptied their pockets for us. People would come over with a tray of lasagna and ten hundred-dollar bills like, 'Here's some lasagna; here's some bread.' We opened an account at the bank just for my medical needs, and it is ridiculous how much people gave. The bankers would call us, all excited, every time a check came in. My aunties made a huge bowling fund-raiser. Hundreds of people came, even the bankers. People donated vacation timeshares to a silent auction. I still get choked up talking about it. How do you ever repay that? You don't. You just say thank you. That money is just about to run out, and it paid for my medical care for the past four years, including the fertility appointments.

"The fertility doctor we saw was incredibly compassionate and explained that eggs freeze well but do not thaw well. As a single, unmarried twenty-one-year-old, I needed to combine my eggs with Mr. Right's sperm to make embryos, which freeze and thaw well. I would have to give myself hormone shots to produce follicles so they could harvest my eggs and combine it with my boyfriend's sperm. At the time of my diagnosis, we learned that I had a clotting disorder, which caused clots in my lungs. The hormone shots combined with my clotting factor would have made me a ticking time bomb and could have killed me; I was willing to take the risk in order to produce eggs. Before I began the injections, they ran tests and discovered that my ovaries had completely shut down during induction chemo. In the end, I couldn't do the shots because I had no eggs to harvest.

"My boyfriend took me to a ring shop with my wig on to pick out engagement rings. Two months later, he cheated on me and broke up with me when I was in the hospital. He fucked me over big time. I was on my pole in the hallway crying into my cell phone. A lot of my family members wanted to have him taken care of. He wanted to be good to me, but deep down, he couldn't handle me being sick. I feel like he left me when I was nearing the end of treatment because maybe then nobody could say he left me in the middle of cancer. My one request of him was that any girl he dates needs to know the truth: that he dumped someone during chemo in the hospital. He told his next girlfriend, who called me saying, 'He can't stop crying over you.' Boo-hoo is all I have to say.

"Thank God, my ovaries shut down. Otherwise, I would have banked my egg with his sperm, and our little baby would be sitting in the freezer right now. Can you imagine what an emotional nightmare that would be? Even though I was having hot flashes and was in menopause, I felt confident my ovaries wouldn't be failing forever and I would have another chance. Day one of my next chemo, I got my period, and I was crying in the bathroom to my mom like

> **"I sometimes feel** that going through love problems is worse than going through cancer. During chemo I snooped in my boyfriend's e-mail and learned he was cheating. I broke up with him on week eight of chemo and have never been so depressed in my life."
>
> —*Melissa Sorenson, 25*

"**I was** a flight attendant and I couldn't fly during chemo because of exposure to germs on the plane. They gave me a position on the ground with all the pregnant women who also couldn't fly. I was infertile and every day I'd go into the closet and cry. It was such a contrast. I was miserable, they were glowing."

—*Katie Smith, 37*

"**I always** wanted short hair but everybody said, 'You can't!' 'cause I'm African American and Chicana and I had quote-unquote good hair: long, curly, not nappy. It felt very liberating to shave it all off. I love my shiny beautiful bald head."

—*Amilca Mouton-Fuentes, 26*

I was twelve years old again. I have never been so happy to have my period. It wasn't until much later that I learned there are online fertility risk calculators, which showed that with my particular chemo, most people eventually get their periods back.

"Preserving my fertility motivated me and my mom to Google 'leukemia' and read every page possible to see if I could avoid getting the transplant that awaited me. My doctor's progress notes always said, 'Poor prognosis, high risk, and needs transplant.' I'm not a doctor, but when I began researching my cytogenetics, chromosomes, and cell type, I knew something was not right; everything I read said I had the best possible subtype. I got a second opinion that said I had a different subtype than the first, but they still recommended a transplant. I made an appointment for a third opinion and visualized that she would say I'm fine; I don't need a transplant.

"I walked into her office dressed in pink, head to toe, trying to look young and vibrant. I had figured out during chemo that I wanted to be a different, noncompliant patient. I was the girl who wore cute jammies, decorated her hospital room, and wore nail polish. I thought setting myself apart from the other patients would make me lucky. I didn't want to be another drab, gray dying person or for my doctors to think of me as room number 5900. I wanted doctors to think of me as Dana, that little superstar who always wears pink. I wanted them to remember I was a young, individual girl with my own disease type and not to lump me into their AML statistics that are based on the outcomes of sixty-five-year-old patients. So I walked in all spunky, pink hat, ready to go, and the doctor told me, 'No, you do not need a transplant.' It was the happiest news. My mom's ongoing heart palpitations stopped, her jaw unclenched. I had to have extra chemo, not that that didn't suck, too, but it was a lot better than a transplant and left the door open for my fertility.

"I told my doctors I was quitting their clinical trial and switching hospitals. Some people have an old-school mind-set that the doctor's word is God's word. I didn't give a shit that I was twenty-one and in theater school. I might as well have been a doctor because my mom and I figured this all out on our own, without a medical background. Sometimes I get scared and wonder if I chose the third doctor because she is pretty and Italian and fun and funky and positive and told me I didn't need a transplant. I worry, What if she was wrong? But I know I made an informed decision, and her treatment plan got rid of the cancer—knock on wood."

> "**As much of** a critical thinker as you might be, once you are inside the hospital it is easy to say yes, yes, yes to everything."
> —*Debbie Ng, 27*

Dana's audacious reign over her care amazed me. Enrolling in a clinical trial can be an aggressive way to advocate for your health, but in some cases, knowing when to quit a trial can be an equally assailing maneuver. Although I had acted against doctors' recommendations on multiple occasions (and lived with the fear of knowing I may have made the wrong decision), I had never been in a clinical trial. I learned through conversations with Amilca, MaryAnn, and

Tracy about the coercion that nurses and doctors sometimes resort to in the clinical trial environment. Every clinical trial has the patient safeguard of voluntary enrollment, which includes the prerogative to drop out at any time, but in a medical climate where doctors may receive compensation from pharmaceutical companies for enrolling patients in clinical trials, arm twisting and biased opinions are plentiful. Dana was lucky. She explained that her trial doctors respected and supported her decision. She continued talking about the difference between life during chemo and after.

"During chemo, I was a super-positive girl, smiling and happy every freaking day. I remember feeling a little embarrassed and asking my mom if it was twisted to be this happy. I started thinking, Happiness is not an external thing. Put me in a hospital bed, a couch, or at a carnival: happiness is inside. I was in a bad situation, but the waters were calm inside. I think that is my personality normally, but it really came out then, and I smiled for a year straight. I don't ever think it was false hope or false positivity, but it was pretty hard-core. I don't know if it was the best way to be happy, but I was drill-sergeant happy, goddamn it!

"When I was in the hospital for chemo, a psychosocial oncologist came to my room to do visualization with me, and I think it really helped me stay positive. (He was adorable, and I had a huge crush on him, so that obviously did not hurt either.) I'm sure a lot of people think it is hokey, but I have a good imagination and I was willing to go there. We would visualize positive things happening to me after chemo. I visualized myself graduating from college, wearing a cap and gown, and walking across the stage. I visualized myself getting married. Granted, I didn't see the face of the man I was marrying, but I still saw the wedding. I saw myself having a baby. I always had to have goals while in the hospital because it meant that I would be alive to meet them.

"During chemo, I was a focused battle girl. You could not stray me because I was so in it. During chemo, I had my mom and that was all

I needed. After chemo was so much harder, and I needed more. The end of chemo was really just the beginning of cancer for me. I felt like I was born again and had to reevaluate my priorities. When I went back to school and started dating, I became flooded with anxiety.

"I attended a really small college, and when I went back for my senior year, all my classmates had already graduated. I'm not shy, I've never had a hard time making friends, and I can talk to anybody but not really about my cancer. I had to explain what happened and why I was there to this whole new group of people who probably didn't care about my life. I made a new friend at school, we'll call her Mary, who I thought was really supportive, but, looking back, I think I was her project. She was like, 'Look at me, I'm so cool for being friends with the cancer girl.'

"Most of my friends from before cancer couldn't handle me 'cause I reminded them we are mortal. So I lost a lot of friends and just started taking more classes. I got to know my professors better, stopped thinking school sucks, and took a genetics course to understand more about cancer. I was the commencement speaker and talked about taking adversity and turning it into opportunity. I feel that is what I did, but it was really, really hard.

"Dating for a year and a half after cancer involves dating men who are very wrong for you and settling because who would want to be with a girl that is obsessed with cancer and thinks she looks ugly? I had a butch do. Women would hit on me, and other people would just stare. When my mom caught people staring and making me feel insecure, she'd be like, 'We'll make you feel uncomfortable right back!' We'd put on a little lesbian lovers act, which was pretty believable 'cause my mom is so young looking. She made me laugh and got me through.

"I became really good friends with Mary's boyfriend, Dan. After they broke up, Dan and I remained friends and eventually started dating. I remember sitting on his bed when we were first together, and I was kinda scared to tell him I loved him, and he was kinda scared to tell me he loved me, even though we both wanted to say, 'Can we just get married right now because we know this is perfect?' That afternoon I showed Dan pictures of me during and after chemo, because even though cancer isn't 100 percent of my identity, there is no me without what happened during that time. He was so supportive, and then he said, 'I have a very hard time looking at these pictures because it hurts me to see you that sick.' It touched me to have him look at them and know he wasn't there during treatment, but it didn't even matter. He still got it.

"When I got engaged to Dan, I felt like my world was crashing down around me because it felt too good. I got so paranoid that I was going to die before my wedding, even though it had been three years since chemo, and my cancer had not come back. It got to the point where I went to see a psychic. Isn't that completely demented?

"Dan and I got married four months ago. At my rehearsal dinner the night before my wedding, I went into a bathroom stall and sobbed my eyes out. I could not believe that this is where I was, at my own rehearsal dinner after everything that I went through. My friend came into the stall and sat with me. I just needed her to be there while I got it all out. It was like I suppressed all of these feelings because they were too big for my brain. It was like, 'Look at where I'm at, I'm alive, I've met this man.' I had to let them out.

"I know that many people who have near-death experiences say, 'Oh, don't be afraid, it is peaceful.' Well, I don't think so. Cancer made me more afraid of death because it made it more real. I am now horribly afraid that everyone I love is going to die. I think Dan is going to die of cancer, my mom is going to die of cancer. Every single person I love is going to die or be taken away. Why? I don't know, just because cancer fucked my brain up. It just messed me up.

"Dan and I applied to go on a kayak trip for couples with cancer, but they rejected us because I didn't know Dan during my treatment.

I was crushed and cried for days, not because I couldn't go kayaking but because they didn't understand that Dan was there for me at the beginning; the end of chemo was the beginning for me. The hard part is starting over again and moving on with life. Dan helped me through fear of recurrence. The thought of recurrence scared the shit out of me for two years. Just the word 'recurrence' made me break down instantly because it would mean getting a transplant. I have been fine and healthy for four years, but I still cannot say the word 'cure' because in my twisted Catholic mystical mind, I think if I say the word 'cure,' I will jinx myself. Dan has helped me with all of this horrible anxiety. He has helped me move on and learn what it means to be a survivor. He has been there at every speech I have given about my cancer. Every event. Dan always says to me, 'Honey, you are taking over the world.' And that is what I want to do.

"Dan is my gift for going through all of this. If I hadn't gotten sick, I would have just graduated and never have met him. I tell him, 'Despite how bad cancer was, if that is what I had to go through at such a young age to find you, then it was worth it.' Some people go their whole lives and never find their match. He makes me happy to be alive. I'll tell Dan a hundred times a day how much I love him because I feel like if this experience didn't teach you to love what you have, then you didn't learn shit. If I love you, I am really gonna love you so be prepared to be smothered, and if I don't like you, you'll probably not be in my life because I have no patience for self-induced drama or bullshit anymore. Dan and I now live with my mom in her townhouse while we save up enough money to buy a house. It is the best thing ever, because I laugh with my husband every day and kiss my mom goodnight every night and constantly tell them how much I love them, even if it drives them nuts."

Dana showed me journals that she and her mom wrote in the hospital. We pored over stacks of photos taken of her during treatment and at her wedding. My own wedding album had been sitting in the corner of my living room for six months, and I had never removed it from the box or shown it to any friends. My wedding had been followed by my recurrence a few months later, and I got a lump in my throat whenever I thought about an image of my wedding happiness frozen on the page. My memories of my wedding day were lush and joyful, but those static images on the page were a graphic reminder that in my life, happiness was regularly interrupted by cancer and the other way around. I could plow through my up-and-down reality on a daily basis, but the thought of revisiting it in full-color photographs drenched me in a feeling of achy sadness. I cautiously asked Dana whether she wanted to see my wedding album. If I started gushing, I wanted to do it with someone who deeply understood why.

RESOURCES

Conducting Research

My approach to kicking cancer's ass was not through prayer or positive thinking but through researching the hell out of my disease. The most proud day of my cancer career was when my endocrinologist told me I was not only a patient expert, but a full-fledged expert on thyroid cancer, and that I knew more about my disease than many of his fellows did. Knowledge is power.

Key Research Tips

Manage your time. Don't zap your energy with an OD of online time. Before you go online, gauge how much energy you have, set a timer, and make a prioritized research list.

Recruit help. Buffer yourself from the emotional weight of sifting through cancer statistics. Give your research to-do list to your geekiest friend or family member to conduct your search.

Use consumer health libraries. These libraries are often based in university hospitals, and most are open to the general public. Can't find one locally? Contact Stanford Health Library for free medical information searches online at healthlibrary@stanfordmed.org, or call 800-296-5177.

Bookmark an online medical dictionary and encyclopedia. Medlineplus .gov is an excellent one. Use the illustrated A.D.A.M Medical Encyclopedia on medlineplus.gov and the Dictionary of Cancer Terms on cancer.gov to help you turn medical babble into meaningful information.

Remember, You Are Not a Geezer

Most cancer research that you will read is based on clinical trials conducted on patients two or three times your age who possess different biological and psychosocial factors. Make sure to read the few reports written just for us.

"Cancer Epidemiology in Older Adolescents and Young Adults 15 to 29 Years of Age, including SEER Incidence and Survival: 1975–2000." You can download this study online from www.seer .cancer.gov. Click on "Publications," then on "Monographs," or call the SEER Division of the National Cancer Institute for a free hard copy, 301-496-8510.

"Closing the Gap: A Strategic Plan." Authored by the Adolescent and Young Adult Oncology Progress Review Group, this report outlines our unique challenges and makes recommendations for strategic change. Visit www.livestrong.org to download the report. (Enter into the search box "Closing the Gap: A Strategic Plan.)

Visit the Young Survival Coalition's Web site at www.youngsurvival .org, or call 877-YSC-1011. This is research headquarters for young breast cancer patients.

Specific Populations Research

Do a Web search for "cancer" and your ethnicity, nationality, race, religion, sexual orientation, geographic location, and other personal identifiers to find support networks and clinical research that are specific to you. Add your cancer type or "young adult" to the search, and see what pops up.

Best Cancer Research Sites

National Cancer Institute, www.cancer.gov, 800-4-CANCER (800-422-6237). Download its articles and booklets, or have free hard copies sent to you. For basic information, choose "patient" articles; for advanced information, read "health practitioner" versions.

Medlineplus.gov. This Web site offers beginner-level, authoritative information from governmental and other reputable agencies and organizations, with easy access to medical journal articles.

Pubmed.gov. This Web site has an advanced database with citations from nearly every medical journal in print. Citations are available either as full text or abstracts (summaries.) When a full-text article is not available through the database, call your local public librarian for help in obtaining a copy through its holdings or through an interlibrary loan. Or inquire about obtaining a full-text article from the Stanford Health Library (see contact information on page 229).

Leukemia and Lymphoma Society, www.lls.org, 800-955-4572. This organization provides extensive research information for patients with various types of blood cancer.

Acor.org. This Web site offers access to more than a hundred mailing lists that give support, information, and a sense of community to those affected by cancer and related disorders.

Checklist for Evaluating a Medical Web Site

- ☐ Displays its logo clearly on each page
- ☐ Makes transparent the purpose of the site and who funds the site
- ☐ Provides evidence-based information from peer-reviewed journals or editorial boards
- ☐ Gives reference citations and the author's medical credentials
- ☐ Includes a privacy policy
- ☐ Uses current information with dates
- ☐ Lists complete contact information
- ☐ Does *not* claim a cure for cancer or promote a treatment with no side effects
- ☐ Does *not* provide patient testimonials
- ☐ Does *not* sell products

Six Tips for Evaluating Medical Studies

1. Who funds the study, and could there be any conflict of interest?
2. What is the size of the study, how are participants recruited, and who are they?
3. Is the experiment double-blind or randomized?
4. Is it original science or a conclusion based on others' research?
5. What are the author's credentials, and is it published in a peer-reviewed journal?
6. Do the author's conclusions accurately portray the results of the experiment?

Fertility and Adoption

Sperm banking by mail. Who knew? Probably not your doctor. Fertility issues are off the radar of many oncologists and physicians. Become a relentless, proactive advocate for your needs, connect with those in the know, and remember that timing is a critical factor for fertility preservation.

Adoption after Cancer Yahoo Group, groups.yahoo.com/group/ adoption-after-cancer. Adoption issues are woefully underdiscussed, underresearched, and underpublicized in the cancer and fertility community. The men and women in this Yahoo group hands down hold the most expertise on this subject matter. Glean information from extensive postings, an adoption agency database, sample letters of support from oncologists, medical forms, and home-study recommendations.

Fertility Preservation Patient Navigator, Northwestern Memorial Hospital, 312-503-FERT (3378). This national service offers free over-the-phone counseling, education on family planning, and assistance in creating an individualized, practical game plan. The first and only fertility preservation patient navigator in the field, it will hopefully serve as a model for cancer institutions nationwide.

Fertile Hope, www.fertilehope.org, 888-994-4673. This is the foremost information hub for cancer patients seeking support and education on infertility, fertility preservation, assisted reproduction, family planning, genetic counseling, pregnancy, adoption, and other related issues and services such as sperm banking by mail. Use its Web site to find a doctor, calculate your fertility risks and options, learn about financial assistance, read published research, and connect with current trials.

Epilogue: Alphaville

I haven't told you about my leaping grand jetés and pirouette turns in my fly-open hospital gown in the hallway of UCSF to coax my barium swallow to slide more quickly down my digestive tract. I haven't told you about sleeping on my friend Mary Lois's living room floor for three weeks when I was too sad to fall asleep alone at my own home. I haven't told you about following the advice of a stranger, an alumnus from my college who heard through the grapevine about my cancer and, although we'd never met, sent me a letter in which he told me to cling to the most proud memory in life whenever I felt overcome with fear. I haven't told you much about my sex life or my work life or my friendships or Shannon or my mom or dad or brother. I haven't told you about the contents of twelve spiral-bound journals that I filled during my first year of cancer. For the first time ever, I have chosen privacy and quietness over airing the details of my life. Instead, I have let others do the telling for me.

Before cancer, my urge to talk about my life was nearly compulsive. I recounted in long storytelling sessions the minutiae of my day. Since I have been living with cancer, there are now swaths of my life that I shelter from vivid words and lengthy descriptions. Twice during cancer, I received treatments that made my body so toxic with radiation that I had to be in complete isolation for four days. I could barely walk, yet I had to stand in the shower and scrub tainted sweat from my skin three times a day. I could hardly lift my head off the pillow, yet I had to change my radioactive bed sheets every twenty-four hours. I did not have the strength to hold a cup, yet I had to drink enormous volumes of water to flush my system of toxic isotopes sitting in my bladder. During those laborious and painful days, I discovered a way of being within myself that I can only think of as preparation for dying. There was nothing magical about these self-discoveries; in fact, quite the opposite. They were moments so unadorned and free of emotion that speaking about them feels like turning them into something precious that they are not. I emerged from the isolation and silence of my treatment realizing that there are parts of living that you hold just for yourself. Parts of living that needn't be broadcast. For the first time ever, I learned that talking about an experience can make it seem more diluted and less real. Those days have made me quieter. They made me want to shut my mouth more often and just listen.

Treatment created in me a desire to listen more and speak less, although I had no clue how to enact this radical change in my life. I felt lost amid our culture's shift from 'cancer' as a whispered word to cancer as a branded, public emblem of strength. I had no role models on how to live with this disease as a quieter, more private experience, while maintaining my stance as an extremely empowered patient. Do you remember Sheila, the woman from chapter 2 who berated me about interfaith marriage, who chose not to spill her guts about her cancer to her friends and coworkers, whom I never spoke with again after our conversation? Of the twenty-five patients I have met in working on this book, Sheila has made the greatest impact on how I now live with cancer. Her privacy about her cancer and her deliberate choices of how little to divulge were an example for me to emulate. Over the course of writing this book, I have followed her lead and spoken less and less to my friends, family, and acquaintances about my internal and emotional experiences of living with cancer. I do not feel pent up, in denial, or afraid to express my thoughts. Instead, it is a great relief to have formed the thinnest layer of ice and ratchet down just a notch or two the temperature of my wild mind and big talk. When I talk about my disease now, I am more intentional about whom I talk to and how much I give away.

In seven years of living with cancer, I have begun to accept that some people simply do not respond to my experiences in a way that brings me comfort. I'm tired of making psychoanalytic assumptions about why they cannot handle my illness. Instead, when it comes to baring my soul about the crap that cancer is, I have learned through Sheila's example to rely on the small handful of people in my life who really get me. I am grateful for the friends and the family members who have endured seven years of this disease alongside me and for the people in this book who have wanted to know about my story, too. Our conversations were much more of a two-way dialogue than these chapters reflect.

Though I divulge less about my cancer to friends, acquaintances, and family, I now reveal my diagnosis to more strangers than ever. Nearly every person in this book was diagnosed at a later, more advanced stage than had we been patients in our fifties, sixties, and seventies presenting the same symptoms. This has created an urgency in my mind to convey the need for doctors, nurses, and the public at large to learn that young adults do get cancer and that waiting to take symptoms seriously can have deadly consequences. The best way for me to broadcast this message is to turn the fact that I am living with cancer into a billboard: I make my message visible but short. If I am at a makeup counter, I tell the clerk I am looking for natural products because I have cancer. I hope she goes home that evening and tells her roommates that she met a woman at work today who had been an otherwise healthy twenty-seven-year-old when she was diagnosed with cancer. I feel useful when I can create in a stranger's mind a very clear picture of a mundane, unheroic young woman living with cancer.

Every person in this book has underscored my belief that the most remarkable cancer patients are not those who are climbing mountains but those who have found a way to climb into bed at night and be honest with themselves about staring fear in the face. It is not the heroic cancer stories available to me on *Oprah* or in *Vogue*, but rather the simple, intimate, nonheadlining stories of the people in this book that have showed me best how to think about, live with, and increase my chances of surviving cancer. Greg Dawson's words are forever in my mind when I am bargaining with my doctors for logical care and arguing with hospital and health insurance companies. "Don't fight the cancer, fight the people who get in the way of you receiving the best care possible." When I hit my limit of navigating the system, Greg's tenacity always keeps me committed and aggressive.

Mary Ann Harvard has become a close friend since we first met two and a half years ago. In phone calls and e-mails, we unabashedly express how much we love and care about each other. We lean hard on each other when either of us is facing surgery, scans, or more treatment. She is on her fourth diagnosis, and chemo is causing her more side effects than previously. She maintains a full-time job as a bank teller, allowing the distraction of work to replace the stress of thinking about cancer 24/7. She confessed to me the other day on the phone that it is getting harder for her to ride past a funeral home or see a hearse driving down the street. "When will that be me?" she asks. When we spout questions like this to each other, neither one of us tries to make the other feel better or happier. Our relief comes from simply talking and listening to someone who will let us be as we are.

Mary Ann's fears are real. With a nearly 75 percent overall survival rate for twenty- and thirtysomethings living with cancer, approximately 25 percent of us will not make it. For this book, I did not recruit a randomized or large sampling of the young adult population, yet this statistic still sadly applies to the tiny group of patients with whom I met. When I last searched online for Wafa'a to find her current e-mail address, the first listing read, "Good bye to a sweet angel of a friend." It linked to an online gallery of hot, glamorous photos memorializing her life as a San Francisco clubbing queen.

Richard Acker's office was next door to Shannon's, and I'd see him when I went to visit Shannon at work. Even with patchy, burned skin and other treatment side effects, Richard never stopped working. When he became extremely ill and I could no longer communicate with him by e-mail, Shannon and I brought a white orchid plant to his house and visited briefly. He passed away about two weeks later. That was a year ago, and his wife, Karen, and I stay in touch through e-mail. The orchid is still alive and is sprouting new roots, she wrote recently.

At the most extraordinary times, I receive out-of-the-blue voice mails and e-mails from Paul, Amilca's husband: when I am driving down Lakeshore Drive on my way to receive a second opinion for a new tumor in my neck, when I come home from a long day of unexpected X-rays and blood tests to address terrifying new symptoms. Paul tells me that Amilca is busy visiting him and their son and influencing their well-being and that she is totally alive in her new incarnation. Although I am not a spiritual person, I do love getting the Amilca update and hearing from Paul how her soul is doing in the universe. He also sends pictures of their son, who is perhaps the most beautiful child alive. The most recent picture is from a trip to Tahoe where he saw his first snow; he is trudging through knee-high white powder dragging a green sled, with a smile plastered across his face.

In my conversation with Greg Dawson, he said he would never put himself through chemo again if his cancer returned. His cancer returned, and he did choose to take chemo again, which caused debilitating side effects. I knew things were bad when my semi-regular e-mail contact with him became less frequent. Two weeks ago, I received an e-mail from his father saying that he had died. I have carried my thoughts of Greg around as a hard lump in my throat. As though part of his very guy-guy attitude has rubbed off on me, it takes the coaxing of a dramatic movie or a particularly cheesy song for me to bawl about him silently into my hands. I want to get a biting and hilarious e-mail from him, telling me what his death was like and whether it matched the experience he described to me when he saw the movie of his life and his bucket of regrets. Meeting Greg once was not enough.

I have stayed in touch with many others in this book, though not closely; they are busy working, falling in love, going to school, and some are weaving in and out of cancer. Nora has climbed her way up the ranks working for a major international aid organization in Washington, D.C. Tracy moved out on her own and divorced her husband. My last email from her included a picture of her relaxing on a cruise ship. HollyAnna studied law, history, and political science in Seattle and then moved back to be with her family on the Yakama Reservation when she received a fourth cancer diagnosis. She still stays busy practicing tradition and culture, riding her motorcycle, and laughing with her friends. Geoff made a solo bike ride from San Francisco to MD Anderson in Houston to raise money for cancer patients who were victims of Hurricane Katrina. There, too, he sat in the halls just being with patients and talking to them about their lives. He continues to be a veteran who places himself back in the trenches. Seth lives and works as an artist in San Francisco. We talk on the phone about writing, art, and cancer, just as we did years ago, late at night the first time we met.

When Seth and I talked this week, he deemed me an expert at waiting, and I think he is right. My doctors have confirmed that there is no cure for my thyroid cancer. I am learning how to live in the skin of the wait-and-watch approach while two tumors nest like eggs on my jugular vein. They still tell me the good news is that my thyroid cancer will not kill me. The bad news is that it will indefinitely bring challenge, pain, and hardship to my life.

People talk about learning to live in the moment. There are times when my present moments shine like diamonds and other times when they are stinger sharp. I think I know well how to live in the moment, and I also know how to vacation in the rich recess of escapist daydreaming. Right now, I don't want the moment. I want to see a future. Some days I feel tethered to a six-month calendar, and I want to see farther and bigger into the distance.

My waiting game looks and feels different now that it is harder than ever for me to cry. I don't know whether my eyes are stone dry because my Drama-Reduction Program has finally worked, because seven years of cancer have cried me dry, or because both cancer and writing this book have made me more used to and less emotional about fear and hardship. Sometimes late at night, when it seems like everyone in the whole world but me is asleep, I curl up on the couch with my laptop and play songs on YouTube that will crack open something in me and release a quick cathartic cry. Lately, I have been listening to "Forever Young" by Alphaville. The phrase "forever young" has a whole new connotation after I've seen people I love die of cancer in bloom of youth. I want nothing more than to grow old in good health. My grandma just celebrated her sixty-eighth wedding anniversary. Shannon tells me we will make it to our sixtieth wedding anniversary. He will be ninety-one, and I will be ninety-three. When he tells me this, I believe him.

Index